Ketogenic Air Fryer Cookbook For Beginners

Simple, Quick and Easy Ketogenic Diet Air Fryer Recipes That Will Help You Burn Fat Forever

Dr. Anna Wiggins

TABLE OF CONTENTS

Introduction

Do you ever feel like no matter how healthy you try to eat or how much you work out; you still struggle to meet your health goals? Whether you want to build muscle or lose fat, or - more likely - a combination of both, it can seem like you're fighting an impossible battle. The ketogenic diet could be the ultimate weapon

The ketogenic diet is named from the process of "ketosis," which is when the body begins to burn fat in the form of ketones instead of carbs for energy. Fat is a much more efficient source of fuel than carbs - especially the refined carbs that most of our diets rely on - and allows for faster weight loss. This book explores the brief introduction of the ketogenic diet, and all the benefits

The ketogenic diet eliminates all grains and processed foods, so you'll be eating a lot of grass-fed or pasture-raised meats, vegetables, and full-fat dairy. You'll find a full list in this book, along with helpful shopping advice. Reading labels is a big part of this process, and learning what ingredients to avoid. Once you know what you can and cannot eat, it's time to actually start the diet, which involves the transition into ketosis

The largest part of the book is, naturally, the delicious recipes. Having really good, easy recipes is crucial to sticking to a diet, and the pressure cooker is the perfect way to eat healthy, ketosis-promoting meals. Whether you're new to the ketogenic diet, the Air fryer, or both, I hope you find this book valuable!

The Ketogenic Diet

The ideas behind the ketogenic diet are not new. This diet plan was actually created many years ago as a cure for epilepsy in younger children. There are even a few popular diets that are modeled after the ketogenic diet, such as the Paleo diet, the South Beach diet and the Atkins diet. While these diet plans are not exactly the same as the ketogenic diet, they use some of the same basic ideas to help their followers to lose weight.

The ketogenic diet is one of the most effective ways for you to lose weight. It allows you to eat foods that will fill you up, without having to worry about gaining weight. You will eat fewer calories, but the foods that you are choosing will help to speed up fat loss, rather than stop it.

Let's start from the beginning. A ketogenic diet is going to be a diet that will force the body into ketosis. In ketosis, the body is going to learn how to burn fats, rather than carbs, as energy.

In a typical American diet, as well as in other diet plans that don't often work, your body is used to working with carbs for energy. The body likes to use carbs because they are easy to convert into energy, but they are not very efficient.

We take in a lot of carbs in a traditional diet. Between eating pastas, breads, pizzas, and even fruits and vegetables, there are carbs around us all the time. These provide us with a nice source of energy through the day, but it is often a high followed by a big crash

When we eat the carbs, we feel good for a little bit. The body has a new source of energy and is ready to go. But the carbs are going to be converted into sugars in the body, which can be extra bad if you are also eating a lot of bad sugars. The insulin will come and take care of the carbs and use them in the cells. But these carbs are usually burnt up before we have used anywhere near the amount of calories that came with them

The result is that we start to feel tired and sluggish. This usually happens within a few hours. And our bodies start to crave more carbs in the hopes of increasing our energy some more and helping us to get through the day. This is a vicious cycle; the more carbs we eat, the more we need to help keep us energized and we gain weight and belly fat in the process

The ketogenic diet is going to try and change this. Instead of following a diet that either leads you to feeling deprived or leads you to failing, it is going to provide you with the foods and tools that you need to get out of this vicious cycle and start seeing some weight loss results.

When you go on the ketogenic diet, you will go through the process of ketosis. In ketosis, you are going to make the body start using fats, instead of carbs, for the energy that it needs. To make this happen, you will limit your carb intake to below 50 grams (fifty grams) each day (some individuals who really want to enter ketosis quickly will stick with twenty grams or fewer of carbs each day.)

Most of your diet is going to focus on healthy fats so that you provide the body with the energy that it needs. Fats are much more efficient forms of energy than carbs. You will find that foods that are full of good fats will fill you up for a much longer time and can naturally lead you to eating fewer calories.

During the first few days of the ketogenic diet, you may feel a little bit lethargic and tired because the body is low on energy and hasn't converted over to ketosis yet. But once that happens, which usually takes between two to seven days, you are going to have more energy than you could ever imagine

The Benefits of Ketogenic Diet

There are a lot of benefits that come with the ketogenic diet. In fact, it is one of the most efficient diet plans on the market for helping you not only lose weight, but to also help you to improve your overall health. Some of the benefits that you will be able to get with ketogenic diet include:

1. Helps you lose weight:

If you are looking to lose weight, then you can't go wrong when it comes to the ketogenic diet. This diet plan is fun and simple to use and will melt off that fat and the weight in no time.

2. Fills you up:

You will be surprised at how much the foods on the ketogenic diet are able to fill you up. If you have gone on other diet plans in the past, you may be ready to go on this one and always feel hungry. But the high fat, moderate protein, and low carb diet is just the thing you need to keep your hunger at bay

3. Controls blood sugar:

Since most carbs are transformed into sugars in the body, eating a lot of them can mess with your blood sugars. And since the ketogenic diet cuts out a lot of the carbs that you are eating, you are able to better control your blood sugar levels. If you are suffering from diabetes or worried that it will become an issue in the future, the ketogenic diet can help to get those levels back on track

4. Clears the mind:

When you get rid of some of that junk you are used to eating, you can actually clear out the mind and make it easier to think clearly. If you are someone who has had a lot of trouble concentrating or remembering where things are, then this diet plan is the right one for you.

The ketogenic diet is one of the best diet plans that you can choose to go on, no matter who you are. Take a look through this chapter to learn more about this great diet plan and then see some of the great recipes that follow. You are sure to fall in love with this diet plan in no time, and the results are unbeatable.

5. Gives you more energy:

Once your body has entered the process of ketosis, you will notice a dramatic increase in the amount of energy that you have each day. You will have plenty of energy to make it through the day and still have some fun at night

6. Helps with your heart health:

Some people are worried about how all the fat content in this diet plan is going to affect the health of their hearts. In fact, it has been shown that the ketogenic diet can help to strengthen your heart, lower your blood pressure, and even lower your high cholesterol levels. This is because carbs, more than fats, are the culprits to these bad diseases. In addition, you will focus your attention on eating the good fats, not the bad ones that can give you trouble.

Foods to Consume and Foods to Avoid

The keto diet urges you to eat. However, you cannot just eat anything you want. In a keto regimen, you should simply eat foods that are low in carbs, moderate in protein, and high in fats.

Foods to Consume:

Berries: You can satisfy your sweet tooth with delicious strawberries, kiwi, blackberries, and raspberries, and other low glycemic index berries.

Vegetables: Eat greens like turnips collards, spinach, and kale. You can also eat non-leafy vegetables, such as broccoli, squash, cauliflower, and zucchini

Sweeteners: Use sweeteners that have the most negligible amount of sugars such as Splenda, Stevia, Sweet'n Low, etc.

Cauliflower: Generally known as the star of dishes, cauliflower is a versatile item that majority add to different kinds of dinners. It can be used for pizzas, wraps, suppers, and with or instead of pureed potatoes. With only 2g net of sugar for each glass, it is not surprising that cauliflower is a champion among the most consistently used ingredients in some low-starch diets

High-fat dairy: High-fat nourishments are a standard part of a ketone weight reduction diet. Fat, furthermore, makes you feel full for a longer period. Some such foods are high fat cream, margarine, butter, and amazing cheeses.

Meats: Stick to meats that have an ideal measure of protein and low carbohydrates; for instance, ground sirloin, salmon, eggs, etc. Eat wild-caught point and avoid farm-raised fish.

Nuts and seeds: Nuts and seeds are crammed with supplements that can empower your body to stay thin and sound. Examples are macadamias, almonds, walnuts and sunflower seeds.

Essential fats: Another incredible source of fats that will fit in your ketogenic high-fat diet is servings of blended salad dressings, coconut oil, etc. Keep in mind that the keto diet is deficient in starches, moderated in protein, and high in fat. A typical ketogenic regimen may have a ratio like this

Fats – 70%; Protein – 25%; Carbohydrates – 5%

The keto diet proposes that between 20-30g net of carbs taken consistently is necessary for the low-calorie. However, if you want to hit ketosis quickly, you may eat fewer carbs and keep your glucose levels low

If fitness is your reason for doing a low-calorie keto diet, then we definitely recommend that you watch your total sugars and net starches. When you participate in a ketone dietary routine and become hungry, you can quench your yearning by eating nuts, nutty spreads, cheddar, and seeds. Do whatever it takes not to confuse your desire to eat with the need to eat.

Asparagus: Asparagus is loaded with vitamins C, A, and K. Furthermore, people think that asparagus can help reduce stress and improve personality stability.

Spinach: It is high in healthy fat and a fabulous side dish. Spinach contains vitamins and minerals, and is heart healthy. It reduces the perils of some common eye afflictions.as well

Mushrooms: Mushrooms have exceptional healing properties. A study has shown that the people with metabolic disorders have seen fundamental improvement within four months.

Squash: Most types of squash have high sugar content, so make sure that you pick the right squash for your eating regimen. The best and most routinely used squash as a part of a ketogenic low-calorie diet is the Summer squash. Summer squash is frequently used as a noodle substitute in dishes; Zoodles, for instance

Avocado: Avocados are actually not a vegetable, but a fruit. However, they can be eaten along with vegetables. Avocado is high in fat, which makes it a major supplier of fat in a keto diet. The half of average avocado has just 3g net sugars. Avocado is the wonderful source of mono-saturated fats, which are important for cutting down terrible cholesterol and triglycerides. It is also a recommended essential food when you have electrolyte issues since it is rich in vitamin C and potassium

Broccoli: Broccoli is a regular food on a ketone weight-reduction diet. It is loaded with vitamins C and K, and what is more, one cup of broccoli contains only 4g net carbs. Critical examination similarly has shown that the people who have type two diabetes can benefit from eating broccoli since it lowers insulin resistance. It also gives the bonus in the form of protective substances that may shield you from disease. Everyone thought of it, as is a staple component of a ketogenic low-calorie diet and, to a significant extent that is correct.

Green beans: Part of the vegetable family, green beans has fewer carbs than many conventional items. Some call them string beans. A cup of green beans contains just 6g net carbs, which makes them a splendid accompaniment to a meal

Kale and lettuce: Used as a component of blended greens far and wide, kale and lettuce are good low-sugar choices. They are, moreover, a beautiful source of vitamins A and C, and can help cut down the threat of heart problems. Regardless of the fact that kale is more nutritious than lettuce, it has more carbs per serving. Consequently, be wary of how much kale you eat in view of the way that sugars are rapidly absorbed.

Foods to Avoid

Fruits: Maintain your distance from and try to avoid such items as bananas, apples, melons, etc.

Tubers: Do whatever it takes not to eat yams, potatoes, etc.

Sugars: Reduce sugar intake to as minimum as possible. Keep away from eating sweets, nectar, maple syrup, even unrefined sugar

Grains: Swear off eating grains like rice, wheat, and oats.

Finding That You Are in Ketosis

How Do You Know You Are in Ketosis? By measuring Ketones. To accomplish ketosis; you need serum ketones in the vicinity of 0.5 to 3.0 mm. The following methods are very easy to utilize. All but one use home packs to measure your ketone levels

1. Breathalyzer: As specified before; when on a slim-down ketogenic diet, your breath has a particular scent. A breathalyzer is a handy way to quantify the concentration of beta-hydroxybutyrate. Remember however that breath ketones can be different from blood ketones

2. Perception: You can likewise tune into your body and decide whether you are in ketosis. For example; when in ketosis, your breath, urine, and sweat announce the presence of ketone bodies, which have a "fruity" odor. If you notice this odor, then, at that point, you are, in all probability, in ketosis. With this comprehension of what happens to your body with ketosis, the next move is to begin on the eating routine

3. Urine ketone strips: Ketosis and other urine ketone recognition strips may not be as accurate because they just demonstrate the overabundance of ketone bodies being discharged from the body through the urine. Be that as it may; they are very easy to utilize and moderate in price

4. Blood Ketone Meter: This is the most exact device to quantify Beta-Hydroxybutyrate. Blood ketone meters can measure with accuracy the level of ketones in the blood, but they are expensive. The meter costs around $40.00, and each test strip costs $5.00. It means that if on the off chance you need to gauge your ketone levels daily; you could part with $150.00

Ketogenic diet Tips

Following the Ketogenic Diet is as easy as counting to three. As long as you have good self-discipline and self-control, you can successfully abide by the Ketogenic Diet. Read the following to know the tips and tricks of following this diet.

How easy is it to follow the Ketogenic Diet?

There is really now profound secret to following a diet except to have **self-discipline, self-control,** and a **vision.** These three main traits are what will keep you on the right track towards achieving your goals – whether to lose weight, burn fat, or maintain a healthy lifestyle. However, it is also true that humans lose track of their goals once in awhile because life happens.

Either you focus on your job and you don't have time to fix your meals or you start your own family and your own goals take a back seat. All of these happen and all constitute and contribute to the failure of keeping track of one's diet. Taking in consideration the happenings of daily life, here are some tips that will keep you on track with regard to following your Ketogenic Diet:

1. Get Enough Sleep:

If you think diet alone is enough to help you shed pounds and build muscle, then you're wrong. Getting enough hours of sleep is crucial to help you achieve the body that you want to achieve. Diet and sleep are two activities that need to be practiced in order to lose weight. A lot of internal changes in the body happen during sleep, so even if you follow your Ketogenic Diet to the key but do not get at least 7 hours of sleep every night (yes at night!), then your hard work will just go to waste.

2. Be Patient - It takes time to lose weight:

Patience is the key to staying loyal to your Ketogenic Diet. The results of your diet plan cannot be achieved or be seen overnight. It takes time to lose weight, especially since this diet plan is not a crash-type of diet. Give it a month or so before you see some changes in your body frame, weight, and disposition.

One way to achieve patience is by being honest and true to yourself. Think of it this way - You didn't attain your current weight overnight, right? So, what makes you think that you can lose it overnight? Gaining may come easy for a lot of people, but losing weight takes longer. Keep that in mind. Give it some time.

3. Hydrate Well - *drink lots of water:*

You need to drinks lots of water to aid in cleansing your body. Your diet in itself is cleansing your body of excess toxins, but in order to wash these toxins out of your body, you need to drink water. Take in at least three litres of water a day to keep your excretory system active.

4. Clean Your Kitchen Cupboards:

Once you decide to follow the Ketogenic Diet, you must also commit yourself to cleaning and freeing your kitchen of foods that will tempt you off your path to a healthier life. Remove items that are high in carbohydrates as well as items with empty calories. Yes, the Ketogenic Diet may have a high fat content, but these are not coming from saturated fat present in junk food. You also need to remove items high in sugar and high in sodium.

5. Weigh Yourself Every Other Week:

You decided to follow the Ketogenic Diet. Yes, you want to see results as soon as you can, but please do not obsess over seeing the results a few days after your first day in. You can weigh yourself but do this every other week only. It is more encouraging for you to schedule a day and time every other week for your weighing duties. Weighing every other week gives you a more positive result than checking every day.

6. Look for a Partner:

There is no other better way to stay loyal to a diet than committing to it with a partner. It is even better if your diet partner is someone who lives with you like a spouse, sibling, or best friend. This way you can check each other's meal plans, help each other during difficult days, and encourage each other to stick with the diet plan.

Ketogenic Diet Mistakes

To drop weight quickly and keep away from weight reduction complications, here are some common food errors to avoid:

1. Consumption of Too Many Carbs: With a recommended body weight of 150 pounds, preferably the largest amount of carbs that you should consume is 30 grams a day. Not until the starches are sufficiently low will the body have the capacity to change from utilizing carbs to maintain your body to using fats for control

2. Being Impatient: Do not go for ketogenic weight loss on the unlikely chance that you will see a dramatic weight reduction within a couple of days. A faultless ketogenic diet is a difference in life style. If you only want to see immediate results, then fasting or starving yourself may be the better (yet unfortunate) decision

3. Too Little Intake of Fat: The human body gets the most number of calories from the intake of substances rich in sugars. If this source of calories is taken away, the body will be famished for nourishment to make energy from. In many cases people imagine that since having fewer starches would be great, so should it be to have less fats, too. This isn't so

4. Comparing Yourself with Others: Each of us is unique even though; our bodies perform similarly. None-the-less, we have individual differences. We ought not to compare our results and outcomes with that of others

5. Not Committed the routine: No one says that the ketogenic calorie-counting diet is simple. The best sustenance programs on the planet don't come without hardships and difficulties. To make a significant change, you need to suffer a little

Most weight watchers who are not completely committed to this eating routine neglect to achieve ketosis and more often than not abandon it after a few days. Try hard not to be like them. When you begin a ketogenic diet, make sure that you put your heart into it

6. Not Eating Enough: Numerous calorie counters neglect to follow the Ketogenic Diet routine, causing excessive craving. Managing hunger is difficult. It is unpleasant and cannot be without much effort, overcome control. Sadly, many individuals who are on a slim-down ketogenic diet don't eat enough, and, more particularly, insufficient fats. Keep in mind that the Ketogenic diet is an eating routine that is high in fat

7. Vitamins and Minerals Can Become Noticeably Deficient: In spite of the fact that the ketogenic diet consumes fewer calories; and it is completely different from fasting, many individuals still confuse the two. Moreover, your ketogenic diet routine ought to be able to maintain your body's health for the long haul

8. Eating Processed Food: The Ketogenic Diet is a comprehensive; entire, and healthy eating routine. Avoid prepared Quest and Atkins bars, and concentrate on eating meals produced using the freshest ingredients. It doesn't mean that you can't eat any prepared or processed foods; just, make certain to keep them to a minimum. Prepared foods additionally tend to have heaps of hidden sugars, so be watchful

9. Consuming the Wrong Fats: Even if the ketogenic dieter eats few carbs; and it is a high-fat regimen, it doesn't imply that you can simply eat any greasy substances out there. Just pick those that have healthy fats, for example, olive oil, nuts, avocados, coconut oil, and others

Ketogenic diet FAQs

When considering starting a highly specific diet, it is normal to have some questions. And any diet worth its salt should provide clear, sensible answers to those questions. So, to help you out, here is a list of Ketogenic diet FAQs, with their most concise answers.

1. Can I go for ketogenic diet if I am vegan?

It is definitely possible to go keto on a vegetarian or pescetarian diet, as any animal fats will provide the right balance to keep you healthy through ketosis. When vegan it is possible, but a little harder work. You would do well to investigate various tasty fat sources and focus on making rich vegan dressings for full leafy salads

2. Can I go for ketogenic diet if I am diabetic?

Ketogenic diets are in fact often prescribed to diabetics as a way of controlling blood sugar levels. However, you can't prescribe yourself one. Talk with your doctor about what is best for you.

3. Will I need to change my lifestyle?

NO, you don't have to, but it will help. You can lose weight by just staying in a calorie deficit in ketosis, and reduce inflammation by eating fewer sugars. But if you exercise, avoid drugs, drink moderately, and make sure you breathe fresh air and take time to relax, the benefits of this diet will be multiplied

4. Will I need supplements?

In an ideal world, no. But if you find that you are having a hard time eating enough fat, protein, vitamins, or fibre, and, for whatever reason, you can't eat the foods you need to replenish them, you might need supplements

5. Will I miss eating carbs?

Of course you will. Whether it's a craving, or you just pass your favourite cake shop, or your friend is eating some pizza, you will want carbs sometimes. That is why we apply the 80/20 principle; so you can enjoy carbs from time to time without compromising all your hard work.

6. How is ketogenic diet different from any other low carb diet?

All diets encourage slight ketosis for weight loss, and all low carb diets dissuade us from eating carb sources. A ketogenic diet is different because it doesn't focus on what you put on your plate, but what you get out of it.

You aren't measuring calories or carb levels, but the physical state of your body. This is a much more intuitive, reliable way of dieting than just paying attention to what goes in our mouths.

Poultry Recipes

Chicken Lollipop

[Prep + Cook Time: 20 Minutes | **Serves:** 3]

Ingredients:

- 1-pound mini Chicken Drumsticks
- 1/2 teaspoon Soy Sauce
- 1 teaspoon Lime Juice
- 1/2 teaspoon Chili Powder
- 1/2 teaspoon chopped Coriander
- 1/2 teaspoon Garlic Ginger Paste
- 1 teaspoon Paprika
- 1 teaspoon Almond Flour
- 1 teaspoon Plain Vinegar
- 1 teaspoon Chili Paste
- 1/2 teaspoon Beaten Egg
- 1 teaspoon Arrowroot Starch
- 1/2 teaspoon Minced Garlic
- 2 teaspoon Monk Fruit Syrup
- Salt and Pepper to taste

Directions:

1. Mix the garlic ginger paste, chili powder, monk fruit syrup, paprika powder, chopped coriander, plain vinegar, egg, garlic, and salt in a bowl
2. Add the chicken drumsticks and toss to coat completely
3. Stir in the arrowroot starch, almond flour, and lime juice
4. Preheat the Air Fryer to 350°F. Remove each drumstick, shake off the excess marinade, and place them in a single layer in the fryer basket. Cook them for 5 minutes
5. Slide out the fryer basket, spray the chicken with cooking spray and continue cooking for 5 minutes
6. Remove them onto a serving platter and serve with a tomato dip and a side of steamed asparagus

Nutrition Information: Calories: 17; Total Fat: 0.94g; Sodium: 28mg; Total Carbs: 0g; Net Carbs: 0g; Protein: 4.89g

Crispy Chicken Breast

[Prep + Cook Time: 25 Minutes | **Serves:** 2]

Ingredients:

- 2 Chicken Breasts
- 1 cup Semi-Dried Tomatoes, sliced
- 4 slices thin Prosciutto
- 1 tablespoon Olive Oil
- 1/2 cup Brie Cheese, halved
- Salt and Pepper to season

Directions:

1. Preheat the Air Fryer to 365 F. Put the chicken on a chopping board. With a knife, cut a small incision deep enough to make stuffing on both
2. Insert one slice of cheese and 4 to 5 tomato slices into each chicken
3. Lay the prosciutto on the chopping board. Put the chicken on one side of it and roll the prosciutto over the chicken making sure that both ends of the prosciutto meet under the chicken
4. Drizzle the olive oil and sprinkle it with salt and pepper
5. Put the chicken in the fryer basket. Cook it for 10 minutes. Turn the breasts over and cook for another 5 minutes
6. Slice each chicken breast in half and serve with green tomato salad

Nutrition Information: Calories: 162; Total Fat: 4g; Sodium: 310mg; Total Carbs: 0g; Net Carbs: 0g; Protein: 14g

Chicken Breasts with Chili Adobo

[Prep + Cook Time: 22 Minutes | **Serves:** 3]

Ingredients:
- 3 Chicken Breasts
- 3 tablespoon Turmeric
- 1/4 cup Sweet Chili Sauce, reduced sugar
- Salt to season

Directions:
1. Preheat the Air Fryer to 390°F. In a bowl, add the salt, sweet chili sauce, and turmeric. Mix evenly with a spoon
2. Place the chicken breasts on a clean flat surface and with a brush, apply the turmeric sauce lightly on the chicken
3. Place them in the fryer basket and grill for 18 minutes. Turn them halfway through. Remove them and serve with a side of steamed mixed greens

Nutrition Information: Calories: 164; Total Fat: 6.48g; Sodium: 330mg; Total Carbs: 0g; Net Carbs: 0g; Protein: 24.82g

Sweet Turkey Bake

[Prep + Cook Time: 55 Minutes | **Serves:** 3]

Ingredients:
- 1-pound Turkey Breasts
- 1/4 cup Slivered Almonds, chopped
- 1/4 cup Keto Breadcrumbs
- 2 tablespoon chopped Green Onion
- 2 tablespoon chopped Pimentos
- 2 Boiled Eggs, chopped
- 1/2 cup diced Celery
- 1/4 cup Chicken Soup Cream
- 1/4 cup Mayonnaise
- 2 tablespoon Lemon Juice
- Cooking Spray
- Salt and Pepper to season

Directions:
1. Preheat the Air Fryer to 390°F. Place the turkey breasts on a clean flat surface and season with salt and pepper
2. Grease with cooking spray and place them in the fryer basket
3. Close the Air Fryer and cook for 13 minutes. Remove turkey back onto the chopping board, let cool, and use a knife to cut into dices.
4. In a bowl, add the celery, chopped eggs, pimentos, green onions, slivered almonds, lemon juice, mayonnaise, diced turkey, and chicken soup cream and mix well
5. Grease a 3 X 3 cm casserole dish with cooking spray, scoop the turkey mixture into the bowl, sprinkle the breadcrumbs on it, and spray it with cooking spray
6. Put the dish in the fryer basket, close the Air Fryer, and bake the ingredients at 390°F for 20 minutes.
7. Remove after and serve with a side of steamed asparagus.

Nutrition Information: Calories: 290; Total Fat: 23g; Sodium: 420mg; Total Carbs: 3g; Net Carbs: 3g; Protein: 16g

Roasted Whole Chicken

[Prep + Cook Time: 50 Minutes | **Serves:** 2]

Ingredients:

- 2 (½ lb.) Whole Chicken, on the bone
- 1 Lime, juiced
- 2 tablespoon Olive Oil
- 1 teaspoon Chili Powder
- 1 teaspoon Garlic Powder
- 4 teaspoon Oregano
- 2 teaspoon Coriander Powder
- 2 teaspoon Cumin Powder
- 4 teaspoon Paprika
- Salt and Pepper to season

Directions:

1. In a bowl, pour the oregano, garlic powder, chili powder, ground coriander, paprika, cumin powder, pepper, salt, and olive oil. Mix well to create a rub for the chicken
2. Add the chicken and with gloves on your hands rub the spice mixture well on the chicken. Refrigerate the chicken to marinate it for 20 minutes
3. Preheat the Air Fryer to 350°F. Remove the chicken from the refrigerator; place in the fryer basket and cook for 20 minutes
4. Use a skewer to poke the chicken to ensure that is clear of juices. If not, cook the chicken further for 5 to 10 minutes. Allow the chicken to sit for 10 minutes. After, drizzle the lime juice over it. Serve with a green salad

Nutrition Information: Calories: 17; Total Fat: 0.94g; Sodium: 54mg; Total Carbs: 0g; Net Carbs: 0g; Protein: 4.89g

Crunchy Drumsticks with Cheese Sauce

[Prep + Cook Time: 2 hours 30 Minutes | **Serves:** 4]

Ingredients:

Drumsticks:

- 1-pound mini Drumsticks
- 1 tablespoon Monk Fruit Syrup
- 3 tablespoon Butter
- 3 tablespoon Paprika
- 2 teaspoon Powdered Cumin
- 2 tablespoon Onion Powder
- 2 tablespoon Garlic Powder
- 1/4 cup Hot Sauce

Blue Cheese Sauce:

- 1 cup Sour Cream
- 1/2 cup Mayonnaise
- 1 cup Crumbled Blue Cheese
- 1½ teaspoon Cayenne Pepper
- 1½ teaspoon White Wine Vinegar
- 2 tablespoon Buttermilk
- 1½ teaspoon Garlic Powder
- 1½ teaspoon Onion Powder
- 1½ sugar-free Worcestershire Sauce
- Salt and Pepper to taste

Directions:

1. Start with the drumstick sauce; place a pan over medium heat on a stove top
2. Add the butter, once melted add the hot sauce, paprika, garlic, onion, monk fruit syrup, and cumin. Mix well
3. Cook the mixture for 5 minutes or until the sauce reduces
4. Turn off the heat and let it cool.
5. Put the drumsticks in a bowl, pour half of the sauce on it, and mix it
6. Save the remaining sauce for serving
7. Now, refrigerate the drumsticks to marinate them for 2 hours
8. Meanwhile, make the blue cheese sauce: in a jug, add the sour cream, blue cheese, mayonnaise, garlic powder, onion powder, buttermilk, cayenne pepper, vinegar, Worcestershire sauce, pepper, and salt
9. Using a stick blender, blend the ingredients until they are well mixed with no large lumps. Adjust the salt and pepper taste as desired.
10. Preheat the Air Fryer to 350°F. Remove the drumsticks from the fridge and place them in the fryer basket

11. Cook for 15 minutes. Turn the drumsticks with tongs every 5 minutes to ensure that they are evenly cooked.
12. Remove the drumsticks into a serving bowl and pour the remaining sauce over it
13. Serve the drumsticks with the blue cheese sauce and a side of celery sticks

Nutrition Information: Calories: 81; Total Fat: 4.2g; Sodium: 157mg; Total Carbs: 0g; Net Carbs: 0g; Protein: 14.18g

Cheesy Chicken Divan Casserole

[**Prep + Cook Time:** 55 Minutes | **Serves:** 3]

Ingredients:
- 3 Chicken Breasts
- 1/2 cup Mushroom Soup Cream
- 1/2 cup Keto Croutons
- 1 cup shredded Cheddar Cheese
- 1 Broccoli Head
- Salt and Pepper to taste
- Cooking Spray

Directions:
1. Preheat the Air Fryer to 390°F. Place the chicken breasts on a clean flat surface and season with salt and pepper
2. Grease with cooking spray and place them in the fryer basket
3. Close the Air Fryer and cook for 13 minutes.
4. Meanwhile, place the broccoli on the chopping board and use a knife to chop
5. Remove them onto the chopping board, let cool, and cut into bite-size pieces
6. In a bowl, add the chicken, broccoli, cheddar cheese, and mushroom soup cream and mix well
7. Scoop the mixture into a 3 X 3cm casserole dish, add the keto croutons on top and spray with cooking spray
8. Put the dish in the fryer basket and cook for 10 minutes. Serve with a side of steamed greens

Nutrition Information: Calories: 321; Total Fat: 13.74g; Sodium: 387mg; Total Carbs: 0g; Net Carbs: 0g; Protein: 35g

Bacon Wrapped Chicken Breasts

[**Prep + Cook Time:** 21 Minutes | **Serves:** 2]

Ingredients:
- 2 Chicken Breasts
- 1 tablespoon Butter
- 6 Turkey Bacon
- 1 tablespoon fresh parsley, finely chopped
- 8-ounce Onion and Chive Cream Cheese
- Juice from 1/2 Lemon
- Salt to taste

Directions:
1. Preheat the Air Fryer to 390°F. Stretch out the bacon slightly and lay them on in 2 sets, that is 3 bacon strips together on each side
2. Place the chicken breast on each bacon set and use a knife to smear the cream cheese on both
3. Share the butter on top of each chicken and sprinkle salt on it.
4. Wrap the bacon around the chicken and secure the ends into the wrap
5. Place the wrapped chicken in the fryer basket and cook for 14 minutes
6. Turn the chicken halfway through. Remove the chicken onto a serving platter and top with parsley and lemon juice. Serve with a side of steamed greens

Nutrition Information: Calories: 297; Total Fat: 28g; Sodium: 358mg; Total Carbs: 0g; Net Carbs: 0g; Protein: 7g

Sweet Chili Chicken Fillets

[Prep + Cook Time: 35 Minutes | **Serves:** 3]

Ingredients:

- 2 Chicken Fillets
- 1 Red Pepper
- 1/2 cup Apple Cider Vinegar
- 1/2 teaspoon Ginger Paste
- 1/2 teaspoon Garlic Paste
- 1 tablespoon Swerve Sweetener
- 2 Red Chilies, minced
- 1 cup Almond Flour
- 1 Green Pepper
- 1 teaspoon Paprika
- 4 tablespoon Water
- Cooking Spray
- 3 Eggs
- 2 teaspoon Tomato Puree
- Salt and Pepper to taste

Directions:

1. Put the chicken breasts on a clean flat surface. Cut them in cubes. Pour the almond flour in a bowl, crack the eggs into it, add the salt and pepper. Whisk it using a fork or whisk
2. Put the chicken in the flour mixture. Mix to coat the chicken with it using a wooden spatula
3. Preheat the Air Fryer to 350°F
4. Place the chicken in the fryer basket, spray them with cooking spray, and fry them for 8 minutes.
5. Pull out the fryer basket, shake it to toss the chicken, and spray again with cooking spray. Keeping cooking for 7 minutes or until golden and crispy
6. Remove the chicken into a plate and set aside. Put the red, yellow, and green peppers on a chopping board. Using a knife, cut them open and deseed them. Cut the flesh in long strips
7. In a bowl, add the water, apple cider vinegar, swerve sweetener, ginger and garlic puree, red chili, tomato puree, and smoked paprika. Mix with a fork.
8. Place a skillet over medium heat on a stove top and spray it with cooking spray
9. Add the chicken to it and the pepper strips. Stir and cook until the peppers are sweaty but still crunchy.
10. Pour the chili mixture on the chicken, stir, and bring it to simmer for 10 minutes. Turn off the heat. Dish the chicken chili sauce into a serving bowl and serve with a side of steamed cauli rice

Nutrition Information: Calories: 226; Total Fat: 8g; Sodium: 486mg; Total Carbs: 2g; Net Carbs: 2g; Protein: 18.27g

Parmesan Chicken

[Prep + Cook Time: 35 Minutes | **Serves:** 2]

Ingredients:

- 1-pound Chicken Wings
- 1/4 cup grated Parmesan Cheese
- 1/2 teaspoon dried Oregano
- 1/4 teaspoon Paprika
- 2 cloves Garlic, minced
- 1/4 cup Butter
- 1/2 teaspoon dried Rosemary
- Salt and Pepper to season

Directions:

1. Preheat the Air Fryer to 370°F. Place the chicken in a plate and season with salt and pepper
2. Put the chicken in the fryer basket, close the Air Fryer, and fry for 5 minutes
3. Meanwhile, place a skillet over medium heat on a stove top, add the butter, once melted add the garlic, stir and cook it for 1 minute
4. Add the paprika, oregano, and rosemary to a bowl and mix them using a spoon. Add the mixture to the butter sauce. Stir and turn off the heat
5. Once the chicken breasts is ready, top them with the sauce, sprinkle with parmesan cheese and cook in the Air Fryer for 5 minutes at 360°F

Nutrition Information: Calories: 180; Total Fat: 6g; Sodium: 520mg; Total Carbs: 0g; Net Carbs: 0g; Protein: 21g

Tarragon Chicken Tenders

[Prep + Cook Time: 20 Minutes | **Serves:** 2]

Ingredients:

- 2 Chicken Tenders
- 1 teaspoon Unsalted Butter
- 1/2 cup dried Tarragon
- Heavy Duty Aluminum Foil
- Salt and Pepper to taste

Directions:

1. Preheat the Air Fryer to 390°F. Lay out a 12 X 12 inch cut of foil on a flat surface
2. Place the chicken breasts on the foil, sprinkle the tarragon on both, and share the butter onto both breasts. Sprinkle salt and pepper on them
3. Loosely wrap the foil around the breasts to enable air flow
4. Place the wrapped chicken in the fryer basket and cook for 12 minutes
5. Remove the chicken and carefully unwrap the foil. Serve the chicken with the sauce extract and steamed mixed veggies

Nutrition Information: Calories: 230; Total Fat: 5g; Sodium: 399mg; Total Carbs: 0g; Net Carbs: 0g; Protein: 18g

Parmesan Crusted Chicken Fingers

[Prep + Cook Time: 1 hour 30 Minutes | **Serves:** 2]

Ingredients:

- 2 Skinlees and boneless Chicken Breasts, cut into 1-inch strips
- 3 tablespoon Xanthan Gum
- 4 tablespoon grated Parmesan Cheese
- 2 Eggs, beaten
- 2 cloves Garlic, crushed
- 4 tablespoon Keto Breadcrumbs, like almond flour bread
- Cooking Spray
- 1 teaspoon Black Pepper
- 1 teaspoon Salt

Directions:

1. Mix salt, garlic, and pepper in a bowl. Add the chicken and stir to coat completely. Let stay for an hour to marinate in the fridge
2. Meanwhile, mix the breadcrumbs with cheese evenly. Set aside
3. After the marinating time has passed, remove the chicken from the fridge, lightly toss in xanthan gum, dip in egg and coat them gently in the cheese mixture
4. Preheat the Air Fryer to 350°F. Lightly spray the fryer basket with cooking spray and place the chicken in it. Cook for 15 minutes
5. Serve the chicken with a side of vegetable fries and cheese dip

Nutrition Information: Calories: 370; Total Fat: 25g; Sodium: 460mg; Total Carbs: 2g; Net Carbs: 2g; Protein: 33g

Italian Turkey Meatballs

[Prep + Cook Time: 40 Minutes | **Serves:** 3]

Ingredients:

- 1-pound Ground Turkey
- 1/4 cup Parmesan Cheese
- 1 teaspoon Garlic Powder
- 1 teaspoon Italian Seasoning
- 1 teaspoon Onion Powder
- 1/2 cup Keto Breadcrumbs
- 1 Egg
- Cooking Spray
- Salt and Pepper to taste

Directions:

1. Preheat the Air Fryer to 400°F. In a bowl, add the ground tyrkey, crack the egg onto it, add the breadcrumbs, garlic powder, onion powder, Italian seasoning, parmesan cheese, salt, and pepper. Use your hands to mix them well
2. Spoon out portions and make bite-size balls out of the mixture
3. Grease the fryer basket with cooking spray and add 10 turkey balls to the fryer basket
4. Close the Air Fryer and cook them for 12 minutes. Slide out the fryer basket halfway through and shake it to toss the turkey
5. Remove them onto a serving platter and continue the cooking process for the remaining balls. Serve the turkey balls with marinara sauce and a side of zoodles

Nutrition Information: Calories: 45; Total Fat: 1.57g; Sodium: 124mg; Total Carbs: 1.94g; Net Carbs: 1.84g; Protein: 5.43g

Jerk Chicken Wings

[Prep + Cook Time: 16 hours 40 Minutes | **Serves:** 4]

Ingredients:

- 2-pound Chicken Wings
- 1 tablespoon Olive Oil
- 1/2 tablespoon grated Ginger
- 1/2 tablespoon chopped fresh Thyme
- 1/3 tablespoon Monk Fruit Sugar
- 1/2 teaspoon Cinnamon Powder
- 1 Habanero Pepper, seeded
- 1/2 teaspoon White Pepper

- 1/2 tablespoon Allspice
- 1 tablespoon Sugar-Free Soy Sauce
- 3 tablespoon Lime Juice
- 3 cloves Garlic, minced
- 1 teaspoon Chili Powder
- 1/4 cup Red Wine Vinegar
- 2 Scallions, chopped
- 1/2 teaspoon Salt

Directions:

1. In a large bowl, add the olive oil, soy sauce, garlic, habanero pepper, allspice, cinnamon powder, cayenne pepper, white pepper, salt, monk fruit sugar, thyme, ginger, scallions, lime juice, and red wine vinegar. Use a spoon to mix them well
2. Add the chicken wings to the marinade mixture and coat it well with the mixture
3. Cover the bowl with cling film and refrigerate the chicken to marinate it for 16 hours to get tasty
4. Preheat the Air Fryer to 400°F. Remove the chicken from the fridge, drain all the liquid, and pat each wing dry using paper towel
5. Place half of the wings in the fryer basket and cook it for 16 minutes. Shake the fryer basket to toss the chicken halfway through
6. Remove them onto a serving platter and repeat the cooking process for the remaining chicken. Serve the jerk wings with a blue cheese dip or ranch dressing

Nutrition Information: Calories: 210; Total Fat: 8g; Sodium: 600mg; Total Carbs: 0g; Net Carbs: 0g; Protein: 20g

Roasted Cornish Hen

[Prep + Cook Time: 14 hours 25 Minutes | **Serves:** 4]

Ingredients:

- 2-pound Cornish Hen
- 1 teaspoon chopped Fresh Rosemary
- 1 teaspoon chopped Fresh Thyme
- 1/4 teaspoon Red Pepper Flakes

- 1/2 cup Olive Oil
- 1 Lemon, zested
- 1/4 teaspoon Swerve Sweetener
- 1/4 teaspoon Salt

Directions:

1. Place the hen on a chopping board with its back facing you and use a knife to cut through from the top of the backbone to the bottom of the backbone, making 2 cuts. Remove the backbone
2. Divide the hen into two lengthwise while cutting through the breastplate. Set aside

3. In a bowl, add the lemon zest, swerve sweetener, salt, rosemary, thyme, red pepper flakes, and olive oil. Use a spoon to mix it well
4. Add the hen pieces, coat it all around with the spoon and place it in the refrigerator to marinate for 14 hours. Preheat the Air Fryer to 390°F
5. After the marinating time, remove the hen pieces from the marinade and pat them dry using a paper towel.
6. Place them in the fryer basket and roast them for 16 minutes. Remove the hen onto a serving platter and serve with veggies

Nutrition Information: Calories: 793; Total Fat: 55.48g; Sodium: 692mg; Total Carbs: 0g; Net Carbs: 0g; Protein: 37.07g

Herby Chicken Thighs

[Prep + Cook Time: 20 Minutes | **Serves:** 2]

Ingredients:
- 2 Chicken Thighs
- 1/4 teaspoon Red Pepper Flakes
- 1/2 teaspoon dried Tarragon
- 4 cloves Garlic, minced
- 1 cup Tomatoes, quartered
- 1/2 teaspoon Olive Oil
- Salt and Pepper to taste

Directions:
1. Preheat the Air Fryer to 390°F. Add the tomatoes, red pepper flakes, tarragon, garlic, and olive oil to a medium bowl
2. Use a spoon to mix it well. In a large ramekin (the size should fit in the fryer basket), add the chicken and top it with the tomato mixture
3. Place the ramekin in the fryer basket and roast for 10 minutes.
4. After baking, carefully remove the ramekin. Plate the chicken thighs, spoon the cooking juice over and serve with a side of cauliflower rice

Nutrition Information:
Calories: 285; Total Fat: 15g; Sodium: 345mg; Total Carbs: 0g; Net Carbs: 0g; Protein: 21g

Cheesy Chicken Schnitzel

[Prep + Cook Time: 35 Minutes | **Serves:** 2]

Ingredients:
- 2 Chicken Breasts, skinless and boneless
- 2 Eggs, cracked into a bowl
- 4 tablespoon Tomato Sauce
- 2 cups Mozzarella Cheese
- 1 cup Almond Flour
- 3/4 cup Shaved Ham
- 1 cup Keto Breadcrumbs
- 2 cups Milk
- 2 tablespoon Mixed Herbs
- Cooking Spray

Directions:
1. Place the chicken breast between to plastic wraps and use a rolling pin to pound them to flatten them out. Whisk the milk and eggs together in a bowl
2. Pour the flour in a plate, the breadcrumbs in another dish, and let's start coating the chicken
3. Toss the chicken in flour, then in the egg mixture, and then in the breadcrumbs.
4. Preheat the Air Fryer to 350°F. Put the chicken in the fryer basket. Cook for 10 minutes
5. Remove them onto a plate and top the chicken with the ham, tomato sauce, mozzarella cheese, and mixed herbs
6. Return the chicken to the fryer basket and bake further for 5 minutes or until the mozzarella cheese has melted. Serve with a side of vegetable fries

Nutrition Information: Calories: 300; Total Fat: 19.01g; Sodium: 580mg; Total Carbs: 0.1g; Net Carbs: 0.1g; Protein: 15.75g

Chicken Kabobs Salsa Verde

[Prep + Cook Time: 35 Minutes | **Serves:** 3]

Ingredients:

- 3 Chicken Breasts
- 1/4 cup Monk Fruit Syrup
- 1 Green Pepper
- 7 Mushrooms
- 1 tablespoon Chili Powder
- 1/2 cup Sugar-Free Soy Sauce

- 2 Red Peppers
- 2 tablespoon Sesame Seeds
- Wooden Skewers
- Cooking Spray
- Salt to season

For the Salsa Verde:

- 1/4 cup Fresh parsley, chopped
- 2 tablespoon Olive Oil
- 1 Garlic clove

- Zest and Juice from 1 Lime
- A pinch of Salt

Directions:

1. Put the chicken breasts on a clean flat surface and cut them in 2-inch cubes with a knife. Add them to a bowl, along with the chili powder, salt, monk fruit syrup, soy sauce, sesame seeds, and spray them with cooking spray
2. Toss to coat and set aside. Place the peppers on the chopping board. Use a knife to open, deseed and cut in cubes. Likewise, cut the mushrooms in halves
3. Start sticking up the ingredients: stick 1 red pepper, then a green, a chicken cube, and a mushroom half. Repeat the sticking arrangement until the skewer is full. Repeat the process until all the ingredients are finished
4. Preheat the Air Fryer to 330°F. Brush the kabobs with soy sauce mixture and place them into the fryer basket.
5. Grease with cooking spray and grill for 20 minutes. Flip halfway through
6. Meanwhile, mix all salsa verde ingredients in your food processor and blend until you obtain a chunky paste. Remove the kabobs when ready and serve with a side of salsa verde

Nutrition Information: Calories: 468; Total Fat: 29g; Sodium: 590mg; Total Carbs: 9.5g; Net Carbs: 6.1g; Protein: 43g

Curried Chicken Cutlets

[Prep + Cook Time: 1 hour 40 Minutes | **Serves:** 3]

Ingredients:

- 2 Chicken Cutlets
- 1 teaspoon Swerve Sweetener
- 1 teaspoon Soy Sauce
- 2 Eggs

- 1 tablespoon Mayonnaise
- 1 teaspoon Chili Pepper
- 1 teaspoon Curry Powder

Directions:

1. Put the chicken cutlets on a clean flat surface and use a knife to slice in diagonal pieces. Gently pound them to become thinner using a rolling pin
2. Place them in a bowl and add soy sauce, swerve sweetener, curry powder, and chili pepper. Mix well and leave to marinate in the fridge for around an hour
3. Preheat the Air Fryer to 350°F. Remove the chicken and crack the eggs into it. Add the mayonnaise and mix it.
4. Remove each chicken piece and shake it well to remove as much liquid from it. Place them in the fryer basket, close the Air Fryer, and cook for 8 minutes. Turn and cook further for 6 minutes
5. Remove them onto a serving platter and continue the cooking process for the remaining pieces of chicken. Serve the curried chicken with a side of steam greens

Nutrition Information: Calories: 170; Total Fat: 3.5g; Sodium: 240mg; Total Carbs: 0g; Net Carbs: 0g; Protein: 22g

Stuffed Chicken with Sage and Garlic

[**Prep + Cook Time:** 55 Minutes | **Serves:** 2]

Ingredients:

- 1 small Chicken, make sure it fits into your air fryer without overcrowding it
- 1 cup Keto Breadcrumbs
- 2 cloves Garlic, crushed
- 1 Brown Onion, chopped
- 3 tablespoon Butter
- 1/3 cup chopped Sage
- 1/3 cup chopped Thyme
- 1½ tablespoon Olive Oil
- 2 Eggs, beaten
- Aluminum Foil
- Salt and Pepper to season

Directions:

1. Rinse the chicken gently, pat dry with a paper towel and remove any excess fat with a knife. Place it aside. On a stove top, place a pan. Add the butter, garlic and onion and sauté to brown
2. Add the eggs, sage, thyme, pepper, and salt. Mix well. Cook for 20 seconds and turn the heat off
3. Stuff the chicken with the mixture into the cavity. Then, tie the legs of the spatchcock with a butcher's twine and brush with the olive oil. Rub the top and sides of the chicken generously with salt and pepper
4. Preheat the Air Fryer to 390°F. Place the spatchcock into the fryer basket and roast it for 25 minutes. Turn the chicken over and continue cooking for a further 10 to 15 minutes but you can check it throughout the cooking time to ensure it doesn't dry or overcook
5. Remove onto a chopping board and wrap it with aluminum foil. Let it rest for 10 minutes. Serve with a side of steamed broccoli

Nutrition Information: Calories: 160; Total Fat: 8g; Sodium: 440mg; Total Carbs: 0g; Net Carbs: 0g; Protein: 22g

Pork Recipes

Sweet Pork Balls

[Prep + Cook Time: 25 Minutes | **Serves:** 5]

Ingredients:

- 1-pound Ground Pork
- 1/2 cup chopped Basil Leaves
- 2 tablespoon grated Cheddar Cheese
- 2 teaspoon Mustard
- 1 large Onion, chopped
- 1/2 teaspoon Monk Fruit Syrup
- Salt and pepper to taste

Directions:

1. In a mixing bowl, add the ground pork, onion, monk fruit syrup, mustard, basil leaves, salt, pepper, and cheddar cheese. Mix everything well
2. Use your hands to form bite-size balls. Place them in the fryer basket and cook them at 400°F for 10 minutes
3. Slide out the fryer basket and shake it to toss the meatballs. Cook further for 5 minutes. Remove them onto a wire rack and serve with zoodles and marinara sauce

Nutrition Information: Calories: 225; Total Fat: 17g; Sodium: 80mg; Total Carbs: 0g; Net Carbs: 0g; Protein: 13g

Pulled Pork Sliders

[Prep + Cook Time: 50 Minutes | **Serves:** 2]

Ingredients:

- 1/2 Pork Steak
- 5 thick Bacon Slices, chopped
- 2 Keto Bread Buns, halved
- 1 teaspoon Steak Seasoning
- 1 cup grated Cheddar Cheese
- 1/2 tablespoon Worcestershire Sauce
- Salt and Pepper to taste

Directions:

1. Preheat the Air Fryer to 400°F. Place the pork steak in a plate and season with pepper, salt, and the steak seasoning. Pat it with your hands
2. Slide out the fryer basket and place the pork in it. Grill it for 15 minutes, turn it using tongs, slide the fryer in and continue cooking for 6 minutes
3. Once ready, remove the steak onto a chopping board and use two forks to shred the pork into small pieces.
4. Place the chopped bacon in a small heatproof bowl and place the bowl in the fryer basket. Close the Air Fryer and cook the bacon at 370°F for 10 minutes
5. Remove the bacon into a bigger heatproof bowl, add the pulled pork, Worcestershire sauce, and the cheddar cheese. Season with salt and pepper as desired
6. Place the bowl in the fryer basket and cook at 350 for 4 minutes. Slide out the fryer basket, stir the mixture with a spoon, slide the fryer basket back in and cook further for 1 minute
7. Spoon to scoop the meat into the halved buns and serve with a cheese or tomato dip

Nutrition Information: Calories: 237; Total Fat: 8g; Sodium: 406mg; Total Carbs: 3g; Net Carbs: 3g; Protein: 14g

Pork Chops with Sweet Marinade

[Prep + Cook Time: 20 Minutes | **Serves:** 3]

Ingredients:
- 3 Pork Chops, 1/2-inch thick
- 1 tablespoon Monk Fruit Syrup
- 3 tablespoon Mustard
- 1½ tablespoon Minced Garlic
- Salt and Pepper to season

Directions:
1. In a bowl, add the monk fruit syrup, minced garlic, mustard, salt, and pepper. Use a spoon to mix them well. Add the pork and toss it in the mustard sauce to coat it well
2. Slide out the fryer basket and place the pork chops in the fryer basket and cook it at 350°F for 6 minutes
3. Open the Air Fryer and flip the pork with a spatula and cook further for 6 minutes. Once ready, remove them onto a serving platter and serve with a side of steamed asparagus

Nutrition Information: Calories: 165; Total Fat: 5g; Sodium: 410mg; Total Carbs: 1g; Net Carbs: 1g; Protein: 15g

---

Bacon Wrapped Stuffed Pork Loins

[Prep + Cook Time: 45 Minutes | **Serves:** 4]

Ingredients:
- 16 Bacon Slices
- 16-ounce Pork Tenderloin
- 1 tablespoon Olive Oil
- 1 clove Garlic, minced
- 1/2 teaspoon dried Thyme
- 1 cup Spinach
- 3-ounce Cream Cheese
- 1 small Onion, sliced
- 1/2 teaspoon dried Rosemary
- Toothpicks
- Salt and Pepper to season

Directions:
1. Place the tenderloin on a chopping board, cover it with a plastic wrap and pound it using a kitchen hammer to be 2-inches flat and square. Trim the uneven sides with a knife to have a perfect square. Set aside on a flat plate
2. On the same chopping board, place and weave the bacon slices into a square of the size of the pork. Place the pork on the bacon weave and leave them aside for now. Put a skillet over medium heat on a stove top, add the olive oil, onions, and garlic; sauté until transparent
3. Add the spinach, 1/2 teaspoon rosemary, 1/2 teaspoon thyme, a bit of salt, and pepper. Stir with a spoon and allow the spinach to wilt.
4. Stir in the cream cheese, until the mixture is even. Turn the heat off
5. Preheat the Air Fryer to 360°F. Spoon and spread the spinach mixture onto the pork loin
6. Roll up the bacon and pork over the spinach stuffing. Secure the ends with as many toothpicks as necessary. Season with more salt and pepper
7. Place it in the fryer basket and cook it for 15 minutes. Flip to other side and cook for another 5 minutes.
8. Once ready, remove and place it on a clean chopping board. Let it sit for 4 minutes before slicing. Serve with steamed green veggies

Nutrition Information: Calories: 604.5; Total Fat: 51.8g; Sodium: mg; Total Carbs: 3g; Net Carbs: 2.8g; Protein: 30g

Awesome Pork Chops

[Prep + Cook Time: 2 hours 20 Minutes | **Serves:** 3]

Ingredients:

- 3 slices Pork Chops
- 4 stalks Lemongrass, trimmed and chopped
- 1 ¼ teaspoon Sugar-Free Soy Sauce
- 1 ¼ teaspoon Fish Sauce
- 1½ teaspoon Black Pepper
- 2 Garlic Cloves, minced
- 1½ tablespoon Monk Fruit Powder
- 2 tablespoon Olive Oil
- 2 Shallots, chopped

Directions:

1. In a bowl, add the garlic, monk fruit powder, lemongrass, shallots, olive oil, soy sauce, fish sauce, and black pepper. Mix well
2. Add the pork chops, coat them with the mixture and allow to marinate for around 2 hours to get nice and savory. Preheat the Air Fryer to 400°F.
3. Cooking in 2 to 3 batches, remove and shake each pork chop from the marinade and place it in the fryer basket. Cook it for 7 minutes.
4. Turn the pork chops with kitchen tongs and cook further for 5 minutes. Remove the chops and serve with a side of sautéed asparagus

Nutrition Information: Calories: 163; Total Fat: 6.68g; Sodium: 202mg; Total Carbs: 0g; Net Carbs: 0g; Protein: 24.21g

Keto Breaded Chops

[Prep + Cook Time: 28 Minutes | **Serves:** 3]

Ingredients:

- 3 lean Pork Chops
- 3 teaspoon Paprika
- 1½ teaspoon Oregano
- 1/2 teaspoon Cayenne Pepper
- 1 tablespoon Water
- 1 cup Keto Breadcrumbs
- 1/2 teaspoon Garlic Powder
- 1/4 teaspoon Dry Mustard
- 1 Lemon, zested
- 2 Eggs, cracked into a bowl
- Cooking Spray
- Salt and Pepper to season

Directions:

1. Put the pork chops on a chopping board and use a knife to trim off any excess fat. Add the water to the eggs and whisk it. Set aside
2. In another bowl, add the breadcrumbs, salt, pepper, garlic powder, paprika, oregano, cayenne pepper, lemon zest, and dry mustard. Use a fork to mix evenly
3. Preheat the Air Fryer to 380°F and after grease the fryer basket with cooking spray
4. In the egg mixture, dip each pork chop and then in the breadcrumb mixture
5. Place the breaded chops in the fryer basket. Don't spray with cooking spray. The fat in the chops will be enough oil to cook them.
6. Close the Air Fryer and cook for 12 minutes. Flip to other side and cook for another 5 minutes
7. Once ready, place the chops on a chopping board to rest for 3 minutes before slicing and serving. Serve with a side of vegetable fries

Nutrition Information: Calories: 376; Total Fat: 8.9g; Sodium: 838mg; Total Carbs: 3.06g; Net Carbs: 0.26g; Protein: 43.9g

Hot Sweet Ribs

[Prep + Cook Time: 5 hours 35 Minutes | **Serves:** 2]

Ingredients:

- 1-pound Pork Ribs
- 2 cloves Garlic, minced
- 1 tablespoon Cayenne Pepper
- 1 teaspoon Sesame Oil
- 1 teaspoon sugar-free Soy Sauce
- 1 teaspoon Oregano
- 1 tablespoon + 1 tablespoon Monk Fruit Syrup
- 3 tablespoon reduced sugar Barbecue Sauce
- Salt and Pepper to season

Directions:

1. Put the chops on a chopping board and use a knife to cut them into smaller pieces of desired sizes
2. Put them in a mixing bowl, add the soy sauce, salt, pepper, oregano, one tablespoon of monk fruit syrup, barbecue sauce, garlic, cayenne pepper, and sesame oil.
3. Mix well and place the pork in the fridge to marinate in the spices for 5 hours
4. Preheat the Air Fryer to 350°F. Open the Air Fryer and place the ribs in the fryer basket. Slide the fryer basket in and cook for 15 minutes
5. Open the Air fryer, turn the ribs using tongs, apply the remaining monk fruit syrup on it with a brush, close the Air Fryer, and continue cooking for 10 minutes

Nutrition Information: Calories 296; Total Fat 22.63g; Sodium 191mg; Total Carbs 3.3g; Net Carbs 3.3g; Protein 21.71g

Roasted Pork Rack and Macadamia Nuts

[Prep + Cook Time: 55 Minutes | **Serves:** 2]

Ingredients:

- 1-pound Rack of Pork
- 1 cup chopped Unsalted Macadamia Nuts
- 1 tablespoon Keto Breadcrumbs
- 2 tablespoon Olive Oil
- 1 clove Garlic, minced
- 1 Egg, beaten in a bowl
- 1 tablespoon Fresh Rosemary, chopped
- Salt and Pepper to taste

Directions:

1. Add the olive oil and garlic to a bowl. Mix vigorously with a spoon to make garlic oil
2. Place the rack of pork on a chopping board and brush it with the garlic oil using a brush. Sprinkle with salt and pepper.
3. Preheat the Air Fryer to 220°F. In a bowl, add the breadcrumbs, nuts, and rosemary. Mix with a spoon and set aside
4. Brush the meat with the egg on all sides and sprinkle the nut mixture generously over the pork. Press with your hands to avoid the nut mixture from falling off.
5. Put the coated pork in the fryer basket, close the Air Fryer, and roast for 30 minutes
6. Then, increase the temperature to 390°F and cook further for 5 minutes.
7. Once ready, remove the meat onto a chopping board. Allow a sitting time of 10 minutes before slicing it. Serve with a side of parsnip fries and tomato dip

Nutrition Information: Calories: 319; Total Fat: 18g; Sodium: 227mg; Total Carbs: 0g; Net Carbs: 0g; Protein: 27g

Tricolor Pork Kebabs

[Prep + Cook Time: 1 hour 30 Minutes | **Serves:** 3]

Ingredients:
- 1-pound Pork Steak, cut in cubes
- 2 teaspoon Smoked Paprika
- 1 teaspoon Powdered Chili
- 1/4 cup Sugar-Free Soy Sauce

- 1 tablespoon White Wine Vinegar
- 3 tablespoon Steak Sauce
- 1 teaspoon Garlic Salt
- 1 teaspoon Red Chili Flakes

Skewing:
- Wooden Skewers
- 1 Green Pepper, cut in cubes
- 1 Yellow Squash, seeded and cut in cubes

- 1 Green Squash, seeded and cut in cubes
- 1 Red Pepper, cut in cubes
- Salt and Pepper to season

Directions:
1. In a mixing bowl, add the pork cubes, soy sauce, smoked paprika, powdered chili, garlic salt, red chili flakes, white wine vinegar, and steak sauce. Mix them using a ladle
2. Refrigerate to marinate them for 1 hour. After an hour, remove the marinated pork from the fridge and preheat the Air Fryer to 370°F
3. On each skewer, stick the pork cubes and vegetables in the order that you prefer. Have fun doing this.
4. Once the pork cubes and vegetables are finished, arrange the skewers in the fryer basket and grill them for 8 minutes. You can do them in batches
5. Once ready, remove them onto the serving platter and serve with salad

Nutrition Information: Calories: 240; Total Fat: 10.49g; Sodium: 640mg; Total Carbs: 0g; Net Carbs: 0g; Protein: 8g

Sausage Sticks Rolled in Bacon

[Prep + Cook Time: 2 hours 5 Minutes | **Serves:** 4]

Ingredients:
Sausage:
- 8 Bacon strips
- 8 Pork Sausages

- 8 medium length Bamboo Skewers

Relish:
- 8 large Tomatoes
- 1 small Onion, peeled
- 1 teaspoon Smoked Paprika
- 1 tablespoon White Wine Vinegar
- 1 clove Garlic, peeled

- 3 tablespoon Chopped Parsley
- 2 tablespoon Swerve Sugar
- A pinch of Salt
- A pinch of Pepper

Directions:
1. Start with the relish; add the tomatoes, garlic, and onion in a food processor. Blitz them for 10 seconds until the mixture is pulpy
2. Pour the pulp into a saucepan, add the vinegar, salt, pepper, and place it over medium heat. Bring it to simmer for 10 minutes
3. Add the paprika and sugar. Stir with a spoon and simmer for 10 minutes until pulpy and thick. Turn off the heat, transfer the relish to a bowl and chill it for an hour. In 30 minutes after putting the relish in the refrigerator, move on to the sausages. Wrap each sausage with a bacon strip neatly and stick in a bamboo skewer at the end of the sausage to secure the bacon ends
4. Open the Air Fryer, place 3 to 4 wrapped sausages in the fryer basket and cook for 12 minutes at 350°F. Ensure that the bacon is golden and crispy before removing them
5. Repeat the cooking process for the remaining wrapped sausages. Remove the relish from the refrigerator. Serve the sausages and relish with turnip mash

Nutrition Information: Calories: 126; Total Fat: 9.63g; Sodium: 631mg; Total Carbs: 0.3g; Net Carbs: 0.3g; Protein: 8.76g

Keto Pork Burgers

[Prep + Cook Time: 35 Minutes | **Serves:** 2]

Ingredients:
- 1/2-pound Minced Pork
- 1 tablespoon Tomato Puree
- 1 tablespoon Mixed Herbs
- 2 teaspoon Garlic Powder
- 1 teaspoon Mustard
- 2 Keto Bread Buns, halved
- 1 medium Onion, chopped
- 1 teaspoon dried Basil
- Salt and Pepper to taste

Assembling:
- 1 large Onion, sliced in 2-inch rings
- 2 small Lettuce Leaves, cleaned
- 1 large Tomato, sliced in 2-inch rings
- 4 slices Cheddar Cheese

Directions:
1. In a bowl, add the minced pork, chopped onion, mixed herbs, garlic powder, dried basil, tomato puree, mustard, salt, and pepper. Use your hands to mix them evenly
2. Form two patties out of the mixture and place them on a flat plate
3. Preheat the Air Fryer to 370°F. Place the pork patties in the fryer basket, close the Air Fryer, and cook them for 15 minutes.
4. Slide out the fryer basket and turn the patties with a spatula. Reduce the temperature to 350°F and continue cooking for 5 minutes. Once ready, remove them onto a plate and start assembling the burger
5. Place two halves of the bun on a clean flat surface. Add the lettuce in both, then a patty each, followed by an onion ring each, a tomato ring each, and then 2 slices of cheddar cheese each
6. Cover the buns with their other halves. Serve with a side of sugar-free ketchup and some turnip fries.

Nutrition Information: Calories: 470; Total Fat: 42g; Sodium: 100mg; Total Carbs: 1g; Net Carbs: 1g; Protein: 22g

Pork Roast

[Prep + Cook Time: 4 hours 35 Minutes | **Serves:** 5]

Ingredients:
- 1½-pound Pork Belly
- 1½ dried Thyme
- 1½ teaspoon Cumin Powder
- 3 cups Water
- 1 Lemon, halved
- 1½ teaspoon dried Oregano
- 1½ teaspoon Garlic Powder
- 1½ teaspoon Coriander Powder
- 1/3 teaspoon Salt
- 1½ teaspoon Black Pepper

Directions:
1. Leave the pork to air dry for about 3 hours. In a small bowl, add the garlic powder, coriander powder, 1/2 teaspoon of salt, black pepper, thyme, oregano, and cumin powder.
2. After the pork is well dried, poke holes all around it using a fork
3. Smear the oregano rub thoroughly on all sides with your hands and squeeze the lemon juice all over it. Leave to sit for 5 minutes, while you preheat the Air Fryer to 340°F
4. Put the pork in the center of the fryer basket, close the Air Fryer and cook for 30 minutes.
5. Turn the pork with the help of two spatulas, increase the temperature to 350°F and continue cooking for 25 minutes
6. Once ready, remove it and place it in on a chopping board to sit for 4 minutes before slicing. Serve the pork slices with a side of sautéed asparagus and hot sauce

Nutrition Information: Calories: 87; Total Fat: 4.02g; Sodium: 121mg; Total Carbs: 0g; Net Carbs: 0g; Protein: 11.95g

Beef Recipes

Roast Beef with Herbs

[Prep + Cook Time: 1 hour 20 Minutes | **Serves:** 2]

Ingredients:
- 1-pound Beef Roast
- 2 teaspoon Olive Oil
- 1/2 teaspoon dried Oregano
- 1/2 teaspoon Dried Rosemary
- 1/2 teaspoon dried Thyme
- Salt and Black pepper to taste

Directions:
1. Preheat the Air Fryer to 400°F. Drizzle the oil on the beef and sprinkle the salt, pepper, and herbs. Use your hand to rub them into the meat
2. Place the meat in the fryer basket and cook it for 45 minutes for medium-rare and 50 minutes for well done. Check halfway through and flip to ensure they cook evenly
3. Wrap the beef in foil for 10 minutes after cooking to allow the juices to reabsorb into the meat. Slice the beef using a knife and serve with a side of steamed asparagus

Nutrition Information: Calories 58; Total Fat 4.36g; Sodium 46mg; Total Carbs 0g; Net Carbs 0g; Protein 6.44g

Beef Steak and Cauli Rice

[Prep + Cook Time: 38 Minutes | **Serves:** 2]

Ingredients:
Beef:
- 1-pound Beef Steak
- Salt and Pepper to season

Fried Rice:
- 1/4 cup Chopped Broccoli
- 1½ tbsp. Soy Sauce
- 2 teaspoon Sesame Oil
- 1 clove Garlic, minced
- 2 teaspoon Minced Ginger
- 1/4 cup Green Beans
- 2½ cups Cauli Rice
- 2 teaspoon Plain Vinegar

Directions:
1. Put the beef on a chopping board and use a knife to cut it in 2-inch strips
2. Add the beef to a bowl, sprinkle with pepper and salt, and mix it with a spoon. Let it sit for 10 minutes.
3. Preheat the Air Fryer to 400°F. Add the beef to the fryer basket, and cook for 5 minutes. Turn the beef strips with kitchen tongs and cook further for 3 minutes
4. Once ready, remove the beef into a safe oven dish that fits into the fryer basket
5. Add the cauli rice, broccoli, green beans, garlic, ginger, sesame oil, vinegar and soy sauce. Mix evenly using a spoon.
6. Place the dish in the fryer basket carefully, close the Air Fryer and cook at 370°F for 10 minutes
7. Open the Air Fryer, mix the rice well, and cook further for 4 minutes. Season with salt and pepper as desired. Dish the cauli fried rice into a serving bowl. Serve with a hot sauce

Nutrition Information: Calories 445; Total Fat 21g; Sodium 374mg; Total Carbs 11.3g; Net Carbs 5.2g; Protein 49g

Chipotle Steak with Avocado Salsa

[**Prep + Cook Time:** 33 Minutes | **Serves:** 4]

Ingredients:
- 1½-pound Rib Eye Steak
- 2 teaspoon Olive Oil
- 1 tablespoon Chipotle Chili Pepper
- 1 Avocado, diced
- Juice from 1/2 Lime
- Salt and Black pepper to taste

Directions:
1. Place the steak on a chopping board. Pour the olive oil over it and sprinkle with the chipotle pepper, salt, and black pepper. Use your hands to rub the spices on the meat
2. Leave it to sit and marinate for 10 minutes
3. Preheat the Air Fryer to 400°F
4. Pull out the fryer basket and place the meat in it.
5. Slide it back into the Air Fryer and cook for 14 minutes. Turn the steak and continue cooking for 6 minutes.
6. Remove the steak, cover with foil, and let it sit for 5 minutes before slicing
7. Meanwhile, prepare the avocado salsa by mashing the avocado with potato mash. Add in the lime juice and mix until smooth. Taste, adjust the seasoning. Slice and serve the steak with salsa

Nutrition Information: Calories 523; Total Fat 45g; Sodium 102mg; Total Carbs 6.5g; Net Carbs 2.3g; Protein 32g

Meatloaf with Tomato Basil Sauce

[**Prep + Cook Time:** 40 Minutes | **Serves:** 5]

Ingredients:
- 1½-pound Ground Beef
- 2 Egg Whites
- 2 teaspoon Cayenne Pepper
- 1/2 teaspoon Dried Basil
- 1/3 cup Chopped Parsley
- 1 cup sugar-free Tomato Basil Sauce, divided in 2
- 1/2 cup Keto Breadcrumbs
- 1/2 cup grated Parmesan Cheese
- 1 ¼ cup Diced Onion
- 2 tablespoon Minced Garlic
- 2 tablespoon Minced Ginger
- Cooking Spray
- Salt and Pepper to season

Directions:
1. Preheat the Air Fryer to 360°F. In a mixing bowl, add the beef, half of the tomato sauce, onion, garlic, ginger, breadcrumbs, cheese, salt, pepper, cayenne pepper, dried basil, parsley, and egg whites. Mix well
2. Grease an 8 or 10-inch pan with cooking spray and scoop the meat mixture into it. The pan should fit into the Air Fryer otherwise use a smaller size. With a spatula, shape the meat into the pan while pressing firmly. Use a brush to apply the remaining tomato sauce on the meat. Place the pan in the fryer basket and close the Air Fryer
3. Cook for 25 minutes. After 15 minutes, open the Air Fryer and use a meat thermometer to ensure the meat has reached 160°F internally. Otherwise cook further for 5 minutes
4. Remove the pan, drain any excess liquid and fat. Let meatloaf cool for 20 minutes before slicing. Serve with a side of sautéed green beans

Nutrition Information: Calories 260; Total Fat 13g; Sodium 617mg; Total Carbs 2g; Net Carbs 1g; Protein 26g

Beef and Veggies with Hoisin Sauce

[Prep + Cook Time: 55 Minutes | **Serves:** 4]

Ingredients:

Keto Hoisin Sauce:
- 1 tablespoon Peanut Butter
- 2 tablespoon Soy Sauce
- 1/2 teaspoon Sriracha Hot Sauce
- 1 teaspoon Stevia Sweetener
- 3 cloves garlic, minced
- 1 teaspoon Rice or Plain Vinegar

Beef Veggie Mix:
- 2-pound Broccoli, cut in florets
- 2-pound Beef Sirloin, cut in strips
- 2 Green Peppers, cut in strips
- 2 Green Peppers, cut in strips
- 2 teaspoon Ground Ginger
- 1/2 cup Water
- 1 tablespoon Olive Oil
- 2 tablespoon Soy Sauce
- 2 medium White Onions, cut in strips
- 1 medium Red Onions, cut in strips
- 2 Yellow Peppers, cut in strips
- 2 teaspoon Sesame Oil
- 3 teaspoon Minced Garlic

Directions:

Make the hoisin sauce:
1. In a pan, add the soy sauce, peanut butter, stevia sweetener, hot sauce, rice vinegar, and minced garlic.
2. Bring it to simmer over low heat until reduced, about 15 minutes. Stir occasionally using a vessel and let it cool.

For the beef veggie mix:
1. Add to the chilled hoisin sauce, minced garlic, sesame oil, soy sauce, ground ginger, and water. Mix them well
2. Add the meat, mix with a spoon, and place it in the refrigerator to marinate for 20 minutes
3. Meanwhile, add the broccoli florets, the peppers, onions, and olive oil to a bowl, mix to coat well
4. Pour the veggies in the fryer basket and cook for 5 minutes at 400 degrees F
5. Open the Air Fryer, stir the veggies, and cook further for 5 minutes if they are not softened
6. Remove the veggies to a derving plate and set aside. Remove the meat from the fridge and drain the liquid into a small bowl. Add the beef into the fryer basket, close the Air Fryer, and cook at 380°F for 8 minutes.
7. Slide out the fryer basket and shake it to toss the beef strips. Cook further for 7 minutes. Transfer the beef strips to the veggie plate
8. Season with salt and pepper as needed. Pour the cooking sauce with a spoon over and serve

Nutrition Information: Calories 190; Total Fat 10.28g; Sodium 505mg; Total Carbs 2g; Net Carbs 1.7g; Protein 18.02g

Worcestershire Beef Burgers

[Prep + Cook Time: 25 Minutes | **Serves:** 3]

Ingredients:
Beef:
- 1½-pound Ground Beef
- 2 teaspoon Onion Powder
- 1 teaspoon Garlic Powder
- 1½ tablespoon Worcestershire Sauce
- 1/4 teaspoon Liquid Smoke
- Salt and Pepper to season

Burgers:
- 1 large Tomato, sliced
- 3 or 4 trimmed Lettuce Leaves
- 3 or 4 slices Cheddar Cheese
- 3 or 4 Kato Buns
- 4 tablespoon Mayonnaise

Directions:
1. Preheat the Air Fryer to 370°F. In a mixing bowl, combine the beef, salt, pepper, liquid smoke, onion powder, garlic powder and Worcestershire sauce using your hands
2. From 3 to 4 patties out of the mixture. Place the patties in the fryer basket making sure to leave enough space between them. Ideally, work with two patties at a time
3. Close the Air Fryer and cook for 10 minutes.
4. Turn the beef with kitchen tongs, reduce the temperature to 350°F, and cook further for 5 minutes. Remove the patties onto a plate
5. Assemble burgers with the lettuce, mayonnaise, sliced cheese, and sliced tomato

Nutrition Information: Calories 421; Total Fat 39g; Sodium 275mg; Total Carbs 3.2g; Net Carbs 3.2g; Protein 21g

Sausage and Egg Casserole

[Prep + Cook Time: 20 Minutes | **Serves:** 6]

Ingredients:
- 1-pound Minced Sausage
- 2 cups Cheddar Cheese, shredded
- 6 Eggs
- 1 Red Pepper, diced
- 1 Green Pepper, diced
- 1 Yellow Pepper, diced
- 1 Sweet Onion, diced
- Fresh Parsley to garnish
- Salt and Pepper to taste

Directions:
1. Place a skillet over medium heat on a stove top, add the sausage and cook until brown, stirring occasionally. Once done, drain any excess fat derived from cooking and set aside
2. Grease a casserole dish that fits into the fryer basket with cooking spray, and arrange the sausage on the bottom
3. Top with onion, red pepper, green pepper, and yellow pepper. Spread the cheese on top
4. In a bowl beat the eggs and season with salt and black pepper. Pour the mixture over the casserole.
5. Place the casserole dish in the fryer basket, close the Air Fryer and bake at 355 F for 13 to 15 minutes
6. Carefully remove the casserole dish and serve warm garnished with fresh parsley

Nutrition Information: Calories: 494; Total Fat: 41g; Sodium: 670mg; Total Carbs: 9.1g; Net Carbs: 5.3g; Protein: 26g

Crispy Spicy Beef Tenderloin

[Prep + Cook Time: 30 Minutes | **Serves:** 3]

Ingredients:

Beef:
- 2-pound Beef Tenderloin, cut into strips
- 1/2 cup Almond Flour
- Cooking Spray

Sauce:
- 1 tablespoon Minced Ginger
- 1/2 cup Water
- 1/4 cup Plain Vinegar
- 1/4 cup Monk Fruit Powder
- 1 teaspoon Arrowroot Starch
- 1/2 teaspoon Red Chili Flakes
- 1/2 cup sugar-free Soy Sauce
- 1 tablespoon Minced Garlic
- 1/2 cup Chopped Green Onions
- 2 tablespoon Olive Oil
- Salt and Pepper to taste

Directions:
1. Pour the almond flour in a bowl, add the beef strips and dredge them in the flour. Spray the fryer basket with cooking spray and arrange the beef strips in it. Spray with cooking spray
2. Cook the beef at 400°F for 4 minutes. Slide out and shake the fryer basket to toss the beef strips. Cook further for 3 minutes. Set aside
3. To make the sauce, pour the arrowroot starch in a bowl and mix it with 3 to 4 teaspoons of water until well dissolved. Set aside.
4. Place a wok or saucepan over medium heat on a stove top and add the olive oil, garlic, and ginger. Stir continually for 10 seconds
5. Add the soy sauce, vinegar, and remaining water. Stir well and bring to boil for 2 minutes. Stir in the monk fruit powder, chili flakes, and arrowroot starch mixture
6. Add the beef strips, stir and cook for 3 minutes. Stir in the green onions and cook for 1 to 2 minutes. Season with pepper and salt as desired. Turn off the heat. Serve with a side of steamed cauli rice

Nutrition Information: Calories 180; Total Fat 11g; Sodium 640mg; Total Carbs 6g; Net Carbs 4g; Protein 11g

Mexican Beef in Savoy Wraps

[Prep + Cook Time: 35 Minutes | **Serves:** 3]

Ingredients:
- 1/2-pound Ground Beef
- 8 Savoy Cabbage Leaves
- 1 small Onion, chopped
- 2/3 cup shredded Mexican Cheese
- 1 tablespoon Cilantro Lime Rotel
- 1 teaspoon chopped Cilantro
- 2 teaspoon Olive Oil
- 2 cloves Garlic, minced
- 1/4 packet Taco Seasoning
- Cooking Spray
- Salt and Pepper to taste

Directions:
1. Preheat the Air Fryer to 400°F. Grease a skillet with cooking spray and place it over medium heat on a stove top. Add the onions and garlic. Sauté until fragrant
2. Add the beef, pepper, salt, and taco seasoning. Cook until the beef browns while breaking the meat with a vessel as it cooks
3. Add the cilantro Rotel and stir well to combine. Turn off heat
4. Lay 4 of the savoy cabbage leaves on a flat surface and scoop the beef mixture in the center of them and sprinkle with the Mexican cheese.
5. Wrap them diagonally and double wrap them with the remaining 4 cabbage leaves.
6. Arrange the 4 rolls in the fryer basket and spray with cooking spray
7. Close the Air Fryer and cook for 8 minutes

8. Flip the rolls, spray with cooking spray, and continue cooking for 4 minutes. Remove, garnish with cilantro and allow them to cool. Serve with cheese dip

Nutrition Information: Calories 227; Total Fat 14.18g; Sodium 485mg; Total Carbs 3.2g; Net Carbs 2.01g; Protein 27.12g

Beef Ribs with Hot Sauce

[Prep + Cook Time: 36 Minutes | **Serves:** 2]

Ingredients:
- 1 rack Rib Steak
- 1 teaspoon White Pepper
- 1 teaspoon Ginger Powder
- 1 teaspoon Garlic Powder
- Hot Sauce
- 1/2 teaspoon Red Pepper Flakes
- Salt to season

Directions:
1. Preheat the Air Fryer to 360°F. Place the rib rack on a flat surface and pat dry using a paper towel
2. Season the ribs with salt, garlic, ginger, white pepper, and red pepper flakes
3. Place the ribs in the fryer basket and cook for 15 minutes.
4. Turn the ribs with kitchen tongs and cook further for 15 minutes
5. Remove the ribs onto a chopping board and let it sit for 3 minutes before slicing. Plate and drizzle hot sauce over and serve

Nutrition Information: Calories 210; Total Fat 15g; Sodium 460mg; Total Carbs 0g; Net Carbs 0g; Protein 17g

Homemade Beef Satay

[Prep + Cook Time: 35 Minutes | **Serves:** 4]

Ingredients:
- 2-pound Flank Steaks, cut in long strips
- 1 cup Chopped Cilantro, divided into two
- 1/2 cup Roasted Peanuts, chopped
- 2 tablespoon Fish Sauce
- 2 tablespoon Sugar-free Soy Sauce
- 2 tablespoon Ground Garlic
- 2 tablespoon Ground Ginger
- 2 tablespoon Swerve Sweetener
- 2 teaspoon Hot Sauce

Directions:
1. Preheat the Air Fryer to 400°F. In a zipper bag, add the beef, fish sauce, swerve sweetener, garlic, soy sauce, ginger, half of the cilantro, and hot sauce. Zip the bag and massage the ingredients with your hands to mix them well
2. Open the bag, remove the beef, shake off the excess marinade and place the beef strips in the fryer basket in a single layer. Try to avoid overlapping
3. Close the Air Fryer and cook for 5 minutes. Turn the beef and cook further for 5 minutes. Dish the cooked meat in a serving platter, garnish with the chopped peanuts and the remaining cilantro. Serve with a side of cauli rice and tomato sauce

Nutrition Information: Calories 174; Total Fat 11.82g; Sodium 232.5mg; Total Carbs 0g; Net Carbs 0g; Protein 15.93g

Fish and Seafood

Cajun Rubbed Jumbo Shrimp

[Prep + Cook Time: 20 Minutes | **Serves:** 2]

Ingredients:

- 1-pound Jumbo Shrimps
- 1 tablespoon Olive Oil
- 1/4 teaspoon Cayenne Pepper
- 1/3 teaspoon Smoked Paprika
- 1/4 teaspoon Old Bay Seasoning
- Salt to taste

Directions:

1. Preheat the Air Fryer to 390°F. In a bowl, add the shrimp, paprika, oil, salt, old bay seasoning, and cayenne pepper. Combine well
2. Place the shrimp in the fryer basket, close the Air Fryer, and cook for 5 minutes. Remove the shrimp onto a serving plate

Nutrition Information: Calories: 80; Total Fat: 0g; Sodium: 370mg; Total Carbs: 0g; Net Carbs: 0g; Protein: 15g

Baked Trout en Papillote

[Prep + Cook Time: 30 Minutes | **Serves:** 2]

Ingredients:

- 3/4-pound Whole Trout, scaled and cleaned
- 1/2 Brown Onion, sliced
- 1 Lemon, slided
- 3 tablespoon Chopped Parsley
- 3 tablespoon Chopped Dill
- 2 tablespoon Olive Oil
- 1/4 Bulb Fennel, sliced
- Aluminum Foil
- Parchment Paper
- Salt and Pepper to taste

Directions:

1. In a bowl, add the onion, parsley, dill, fennel, and garlic. Mix and drizzle the olive oil over it
2. Preheat the Air Fryer to 350°F. Open the cavity of the fish and fill with the fennel mixture
3. Wrap the fish completely in parchment paper and then in foil
4. Place the fish in the fryer basket and cook it for 10 minutes
5. Remove the paper and foil and top with lemon slices. Serve with a side of cooked mushrooms.

Nutrition Information:

Calories: 43; Total Fat: 2.11g; Sodium: 84mg; Total Carbs: 0.09g; Net Carbs: 0.09g; Protein: 5.61g

Fried Catfish Fillets

[Prep + Cook Time: 40 Minutes | **Serves:** 2]

Ingredients:

- 2 Catfish Fillets
- 3 tablespoon Keto Breadcrumbs
- 2 sprigs Parsley, chopped
- 1 teaspoon dry Fish Seasoning, of choice
- 1 teaspoon Cayenne Pepper
- Olive Oil Cooking Spray
- Salt to taste, optional

Directions:

1. Preheat Air Fryer to 400°F. Meanwhile, pour all the dry ingredients except the parsley in a zipper bag
2. Pat dry and add the fish pieces. Close the bag and shake to coat the fish well. Do this with one fish piece at a time
3. Lightly spray the fish with olive oil. Arrange them in the fryer basket, one at a time depending on the size of the fish.
4. Close the Air Fryer and cook for 10 minutes. Flip the fish and cook further for 10 minutes

5. For extra crispiness, cook further for 3 minutes. Garnish with parsley and serve as a lunch accompaniment

Nutrition Information: Calories: 182; Total Fat: 12.8g; Sodium: 79mg; Total Carbs: 1g; Net Carbs: 0.8g; Protein: 11.12g

Keto Seafood Pie

[Prep + Cook Time: 60 Minutes | **Serves:** 2]

Ingredients:

- 1-pound Turnips, peeled and quartered
- 1 Carrot, grated
- 1 cup Seafood Marinara Mix
- 1/2 head Baby Fennel, grated
- 1/2 Lemon, juiced
- 2 tablespoon Butter
- 1 tablespoon Milk
- A handful Baby Spinach
- 1 small Tomato, diced
- 1/2 Celery Sticks, grated
- 1 bunch Dill Sprigs, chopped
- 1 sprig Parsley, chopped
- 1 cup Water
- 1 small red Chili, minced
- 1/2 cup grated Cheddar Cheese
- Salt and Pepper to taste

Directions:

1. Pour the turnips into a pan, add the water, and bring it to a boil over medium heat on a stove top. Use a fork to check that it is soft and mash-able, after about 12 minutes. Drain the water and use a potato masher to mash it
2. Add the butter, milk, salt, and pepper. Mash until smooth and well mixed. Set aside
3. In a bowl, add the celery, carrots, cheese, chili, fennel, parsley, lemon juice, seafood mix, dill, tomato, spinach, salt, and pepper. Mix well. Preheat the Air Fryer to 330°F. In a 15 cm casserole dish, add half of the carrots mixture and level it. Top with half of the turnip mixture and level it
4. Place the dish in the Air Fryer and bake for 20 minutes ensuring that the mash is golden brown and the seafood is properly cooked
5. Remove the dish and add the remaining seafood mixture and level it out. Top with the remaining turnip mash and level it too. Place the dish back into the Air Fryer and cook at 330°F for 20 more minutes
6. Once ready ensuring that it is well cooked, remove the dish. Slice the pie and serve with a green salad

Nutrition Information: Calories: 318; Total Fat: 22.55g; Sodium: 617mg; Total Carbs: 3.3g; Net Carbs: 2.27g; Protein: 24.6g

Crispy Prawn in Bacon

[Prep + Cook Time: 35 Minutes | **Serves:** 3]

Ingredients:

- 8 Bacon Slices
- Lemon Wedges for garnishing
- 8 Jumbo Prawns, peeled and deveined
- Toothpicks

Directions:

1. Wrap each prawn from head to tail with each bacon slice overlapping to keep the bacon in place.
2. Secure the end of the bacon with toothpick. It's ok not to cover the ends of the cheese with bacon
3. Refrigerate for 15 minutes.
4. Preheat the Air Fryer to 400°F. Arrange the bacon wrapped prawns in the fryer's basket
5. Close the Air Fryer and cook for 7 minutes or until the bacon has browned and crispy
6. Transfer prawns unto a paper towel to cool for 2 minutes
7. Remove the toothpicks and serve the bacon wrapped prawns with lemon wedges and a side of steamed green vegetables

Nutrition Information: Calories: 33; Total Fat: 2.19g; Sodium: 144mg; Total Carbs: 0.12g; Net Carbs: 0.12g; Protein: 3.06g

Crab Croquettes

[**Prep + Cook Time:** 40 Minutes | **Serves:** 5]

Ingredients:

Filling:

- 1½-pound Lump Crab Meat
- 2½ tbsp. chopped Celery
- 1/2 teaspoon chopped Chives
- 3 Egg Whites, beaten
- 1/3 cup Sour Cream
- 1/3 cup Mayonnaise

- 1 Red Pepper, chopped finely
- 1/3 cup chopped Red Onion
- 1 teaspoon chopped Parsley
- 1 teaspoon Cayenne Pepper
- 1½ tablespoon Olive Oil
- 1/2 teaspoon chopped Tarragon

Breading:

- 1½ cup Keto Breadcrumbs
- 2 teaspoon Olive Oil
- 4 Eggs, beaten

- 1 cup Almond Flour
- Salt to taste

Directions:

1. Place a skillet over medium heat on a stove top, add 1½ tablespoon olive oil, red pepper, onion, and celery. Sauté for 5 minutes or until sweaty and translucent. Turn off heat. Add the breadcrumbs, remaining olive oil, and salt to a food processor. Blend to mix evenly. Set aside
2. In two separate bowls, add the almond flour and 4 eggs respectively. Set aside
3. In a separate mixing bowl, add the crab meat, mayonnaise, egg whites, sour cream, tarragon, chives, parsley, cayenne pepper, and the celery sauté and mix evenly. Form bite-size balls from the mixture and place into a plate
4. Preheat the Air Fryer to 390°F. Dip each crab meatball (croquettes) in the eggs mixture and press them in the breadcrumb mixture. Place the croquettes in the fryer basket, 12 to 15 at a time. Avoid overcrowding.
5. Close the Air Fryer and cook for 10 minutes or until golden brown
6. Remove them and plate them. Serve the crab croquettes with tomato dipping sauce and a side of vegetable fries

Nutrition Information: Calories: 106; Total Fat: 5.03g; Sodium: 217mg; Total Carbs: 0.42g; Net Carbs: 0.41g; Protein: 14g

Baby Octopus Salad

[**Prep + Cook Time:** 55 Minutes | **Serves:** 2]

Ingredients:

- 1-pound Baby Octopus, thoroughly cleaned
- 1 medium Red Onion, sliced
- 1 small bunch Baby Fennel, chopped
- 1 cup semi-dried Tomatoes, chopped
- 2 handfuls Arugula
- 1 small bunch Parsley, chopped roughly
- 1½ tablespoon Capers

- 1 ¼ tbsp. Balsamic Glaze
- 1/4 cup chopped Grilled Halloumi
- 1½ tbsp. Olive Oil
- 2 cloves Garlic, minced
- 1 long Red Chili, minced
- 1½ cups Water
- Salt and Pepper to taste

Directions:

1. Pour the water in a pot and bring it to boil over medium heat on a stove top
2. Cut the octopus into bite sizes and add it to the boiling water for 45 seconds. Drain the water. Add the garlic, olive oil, and octopus in a bowl. Coat the octopus with the garlic and olive oil. Leave it to marinate for 20 minutes
3. Preheat the Air Fryer to 390°F. Place the octopus in the fryer basket and grill it for 5 minutes
4. Meanwhile, in a salad mixing bowl, add the capers, halloumi, chili, tomatoes, olives, parsley, red onion, fennel, octopus, arugula, and balsamic glaze

5. Season with salt and pepper and mix. Serve with a side of keto toasts

Nutrition Information: Calories: 299; Total Fat: 20.84g; Sodium: 232mg; Total Carbs: 3g; Net Carbs: 3.4g; Protein: 17.37g

Grilled Barramundi

[**Prep + Cook Time:** 35 Minutes | **Serves:** 3]

Ingredients:
- 3 (½ lb.) Barramundi Fillets
- 6-ounce Unsalted Butter
- 2 Bay Leaves
- 15 Black Peppercorns
- 2 cloves Garlic, minced
- 3/4 cup Thickened Cream
- 1/2 cup White Wine
- 2 Lemons, juiced
- 2 Shallots, chopped
- Salt and Pepper to taste

Directions:
1. Preheat the Air Fryer to 390°F. Place the barramundi fillets on a baking paper and put them in the fryer basket.
2. Close the Air Fryer and grill for 15 minutes. After 15 minutes, remove them and put them on a serving platter without the baking paper
3. Place a small pan over low heat on a stove top. Add the garlic and shallots, and dry fry for a few seconds
4. Add the wine, bay leaves, and peppercorns. Stir and allow the liquid reduce by three quarters
5. Add the cream. Stir and let the sauce thicken into a dark cream color.
6. Add the butter, whisk it into the cream until it has fully melted
7. Add the lemon juice, pepper, and salt. Turn the heat off. Strain the sauce into a serving bowl.
8. Pour the sauce over the fish. Serve with a side of cauli rice

Nutrition Information: Calories: 155; Total Fat: 4.33g; Sodium: 392mg; Total Carbs: 0.81g; Net Carbs: 0.81g; Protein: 25.53g

Greek Salmon with Dill Sauce

[**Prep + Cook Time:** 25 Minutes | **Serves:** 4]

Ingredients:
- 4 (6-oz) Salmon Pieces
- 2 teaspoon Olive Oil
- 3 tablespoon chopped Dill + extra for garnishing
- 1 cup Sour Cream
- 1 cup Greek Yoghurt, full fat
- Salt and Pepper to taste

Directions:
1. Make the dill sauce: in a bowl, add the sour cream, yogurt, dill, and salt. Mix it well
2. Preheat the Air Fryer to 270°F. Drizzle the olive oil over the salmon. Season with salt and pepper. Rub lightly with your hands.
3. Arrange the salmon pieces in the fryer basket and cook them for 15 minutes
4. Remove the salmon onto the serving platter and top with dill sauce. Serve with steamed asparagus

Nutrition Information: Calories: 240; Total Fat: 6g; Sodium: 690mg; Total Carbs: 0g; Net Carbs: 0g; Protein: 16g

Cod Fish Nuggets

[Prep + Cook Time: 20 Minutes | **Serves:** 2]

Ingredients:

- 4 Cod Fillets
- 2 tablespoon Olive Oil
- 2 Eggs, beaten
- 1 cup Almond Flour
- 1 cup Keto Breadcrumbs
- A pinch of Salt

Directions:

1. Preheat the Air Fryer to 390°F. Place the breadcrumbs, olive oil, and salt in a food processor and process until evenly combined
2. Pour the breadcrumb mixture into a bowl, the eggs into another bowl, and the flour into a third bowl
3. Toss the cod fillets in the almond flour, then in the eggs, and then in the breadcrumb mixture
4. Place them in the fryer basket, close the Air Fryer, and cook for 9 minutes. At the 5-minute mark, quickly turn the chicken nuggets over.
5. Once golden brown, remove onto a serving plate and serve with vegetable fries

Nutrition Information: Calories: 168; Total Fat: 7.57g; Sodium: 399mg; Total Carbs: 0.14g; Net Carbs: 0.14g; Protein: 16.68g

Snacks and Appetizers

Keto Cheese Balls

[**Prep + Cook Time:** 50 Minutes | **Serves:** 4]

Ingredients:

- 2 cups crumbled Cottage Cheese
- 1 cup Almond Flour
- 1 medium Onion, finely chopped
- 1 Green Chili, finely chopped
- 1 cup Keto Breadcrumbs
- 2 cups grated Parmesan Cheese
- 2 Turnips, peeled and chopped
- 1½ teaspoon Red Chili Flakes
- 4 tablespoon chopped Coriander Leaves
- Water
- Salt to taste

Directions:

1. Place the turnips in a pot, add water and bring them to boil over medium heat on a stove top for 25 to 30 minutes until soft
2. Turn off the heat, drain the turnips through a sieve, and place in a bowl. With a potato masher, mash the turnips and leave to cool
3. Now, add the cottage cheese, parmesan cheese, onion, red chili flakes, green chili, salt, coriander, and almond flour to the turnip mash
4. Use a wooden spoon to mix the ingredients well, then, use your hands to mold out bite-size balls. Pour the breadcrumbs in a bowl and roll each cheese ball lightly in it. Place them on a tray
5. Preheat Air Fryer to 350°F. Open the Air Fryer and place 8 to 10 cheese balls in the fryer basket. Close the Air Fryer and cook them for 15 minutes. Once ready, remove them to a plate
6. Repeat the cooking process for the remaining cheese balls. Serve with tomato-based dip

Nutrition Information: Calories 150; Total Fat 9g; Sodium 260mg; Total Carbs 5g; Net Carbs 5g; Protein 3g

French Toast Sticks

[**Prep + Cook Time:** 13 Minutes | **Serves:** 3]

Ingredients:

- 5 slices Keto Bread
- 1½ tablespoon Butter
- 1/8 teaspoon Cinnamon Powder
- 3 Eggs
- A pinch Nutmeg Powder
- A pinch Clove Powder
- Cooking Spray
- Salt and Pepper to taste

Directions:

1. Preheat the Air Fryer to 350°F. In a bowl, add the clove powder, eggs, nutmeg powder, cinnamon powder.
2. Beat well using a whisk. Use a bread knife to apply butter on both sides of the bread slices and cut them into 3 or 4 strips (depending on the size of the slice)
3. Dip each strip in the egg mixture and arrange them in one layer in the fryer basket. Cook for 2 minutes.
4. Once ready, pull out the fryer basket and spray the toasts with cooking spray. Flip the toasts and spray the other side with cooking spray.
5. Slide the fryer basket back into the Air Fryer and continue cooking for 4 minutes
6. Keep a constant eye on the toasts to prevent them from burning
7. Once the toasts are golden brown, remove them onto a serving platter. Dust with cinnamon and serve with sugar-free syrup

Nutrition Information: Calories: 76; Total Fat: 4.33g; Sodium: 74mg; Total Carbs: 3.4g; Net Carbs: 3g; Protein: 2.23g

Cheese Sticks

Ingredients:

- 2 tablespoon Butter
- 6 (6 oz) Bread Cheese

Directions:

1. Put the butter in a small bowl and melt it in the microwave, for about 2 minutes. Remove it and set aside
2. With a knife, cut the cheese into equal sized sticks. Brush each stick with butter. Arrange the coated cheese sticks in a single layer on the fryer basket
3. Slide in the fryer basket and cook at 390°F 10 minutes. Flip them halfway to brown evenly. Serve with a tomato dip

Nutrition Information: Calories 112; Total Fat 10g; Sodium 155mg; Total Carbs 1g; Net Carbs 1g; Protein 6g

Breaded Button Mushrooms

Ingredients:

- 1-pound small Button Mushrooms, well cleaned
- 2 cups Keto Breadcrumbs
- 2 Eggs, beaten
- 2 cups Parmigiano Reggiano Cheese, grated
- Salt and Pepper to taste

Directions:

1. Preheat the Air Fryer to 360°F
2. Pour the breadcrumbs in a bowl, add the salt and pepper and mix well.
3. Pour the cheese in a bowl and set aside
4. Dip each mushroom in the eggs, then in the breadcrumbs, and then in the cheese.
5. Slide out the fryer basket and add 6 to 10 mushrooms to it
6. Close the Air Fryer and cook them for 20 minutes
7. Once ready, remove onto a serving platter and repeat the cooking process for the remaining mushrooms. Serve with cheese dip

Nutrition Information: Calories 24; Total Fat 0.4g; Sodium 380mg; Total Carbs 3.3g; Net Carbs 2.3g; Protein 3.1g

Calamari and Olives

Ingredients:

- 1/2-pound Calamari Rings
- 2 strips Chili Pepper, chopped
- 1 tablespoon Olive Oil
- 1/2-piece Coriander, chopped
- 1 cup Pimiento Stuffed Green Olives, sliced
- Salt and Black Pepper to taste

Directions:

1. In a bowl, add the calamari rings, chili pepper, salt, black pepper, oil, and coriander. Mix and leave the calamari to marinate for 10 minutes
2. Pour the calamari into an oven-safe bowl, good enough to fit into the fryer basket
3. Slide the fryer basket out, place the bowl in it, and slide the basket back in
4. Cook the calamari for 15 minutes stirring every 5 minutes using a spoon
5. After 15 minutes, open the Air Fryer, and add the olives.
6. Stir, close the Air Fryer and continue cooking for 3 minutes
7. Once ready, transfer to a serving platter. Serve warm with a side of keto bread slices.

Nutrition Information: Calories 128; Total Fat 1.92g; Sodium 514mg; Total Carbs 0g; Net Carbs 0g; Protein 21.63g

Parmesan Crusted Pickles

[Prep + Cook Time: 35 Minutes | **Serves:** 4]

Ingredients:

- 3 cups Large Dill Pickles, sliced in 1/4 - inches
- 1 cup Grated Parmesan Cheese
- 2 teaspoon Water
- 1½ cup Keto Breadcrumbs, smooth
- 2 Eggs
- Black Pepper to taste
- Cooking Spray

Directions:

1. Add the breadcrumbs and black pepper to a bowl and mix well. Set aside
2. In another bowl, crack the eggs and beat with the water. Set aside. Add the cheese to a separate bowl. Set aside
3. Line a flat surface with a paper towel and arrange the pickle slices on it to extra as much water from them. Preheat the Air Fryer to 400°F.
4. Pull out the fryer basket and spray it lightly with cooking spray
5. Dredge the pickle slices it in the egg mixture, then in breadcrumbs and then in cheese
6. Pull out the fryer basket and lay as much coated pickle slices in it without overlapping. Slide the fryer basket back in and cook for 4 minutes
7. Open the Air Fryer and turn the pickles over. Cook further for 4 to 5 minutes to make them crispy. Once ready, remove onto a serving platter and serve with a cheese dip

Nutrition Information: Calories 13; Total Fat 2g; Sodium 833mg; Total Carbs 1g; Net Carbs 0.2g; Protein 1g

Chicken and Bacon Wrapped Jalapenos

[Prep + Cook Time: 35 Minutes | **Serves:** 4]

Ingredients:

- 4 Chicken Breasts, butterflied and halved
- 8 Jalapeno Peppers, halved lengthwise and seeded
- 16 slices Turkey or Pork Bacon
- 1 cup Keto Breadcrumbs
- 2 Eggs
- 6-ounce Cheddar Cheese
- 6-ounce Cream Cheese
- Cooking Spray
- Salt and Pepper to taste

Directions:

1. Wrap the chicken in cling film and place on a chopping board. Using a rolling pin, pound the chicken evenly to flatten them but not too thin
2. Afterward, remove the cling film and season the chicken with pepper and salt on both sides. In a bowl, add the cream cheese, cheddar cheese, a pinch each of pepper, and salt. Mix well. Take each jalapeno and spoon in the cheese mixture to the brim
3. Now, on a chopping board, flatten each piece of chicken and lay two bacon slices each on them. Place a stuffed jalapeno on each laid out chicken and bacon set and wrap the jalapenos in them. Place aside
4. Preheat the Air Fryer to 350°F. Add the eggs to a bowl and pour the breadcrumbs in another bowl. Also, set a flat plate aside.
5. Take each wrapped jalapeno and dip it into the eggs and then thoroughly in the breadcrumbs. Place them on the flat plate.
6. Open the Air Fryer and lightly grease the fryer basket with cooking spray
7. Arrange 4 to 5 breaded jalapenos in the fryer basket, close the Air Fryer and cook for 7 minutes. Prepare a paper towel lined plate and set aside.
8. Once the timer beeps, open the Air Fryer, turn the jalapenos, close and cook further for 4 minutes
9. Once ready, remove them onto the paper towel lined plate and repeat the cooking process for the remaining jalapenos. Serve with a sweet dip for an enhanced taste

Nutrition Information: Calories 204; Total Fat 12.8g; Sodium 206mg; Total Carbs 3g; Net Carbs 1.7g; Protein 9.26g

Beef Meatballs

[Prep + Cook Time: 25 Minutes | **Serves:** 2 to 3]

Ingredients:

- 1/2-pound Ground Beef
- 1 small finger Ginger, crushed
- 1/4 teaspoon Dry Mustard
- 1 tablespoon Hot Sauce
- 3 tablespoon Vinegar
- 1/2 cup Tomato Ketchup, reduced sugar
- 2 tablespoon Monk Fruit Sugar
- 1½ teaspoon Lemon Juice
- Salt and Pepper to taste, if needed

Directions:

1. In a bowl, add the beef, ginger, hot sauce, vinegar, lemon juice, tomato ketchup, monk fruit sugar, dry mustard, pepper, and salt and mix well using a spoon
2. Mold out 2-inch sized balls out of the mixture using your hands
3. Pull out the fryer basket and add the balls to it without overcrowding
4. Slide the fryer basket back in and cook the balls at 370°F for 15 minutes
5. Remove them onto a serving platter and repeat the frying process for any remaining balls. Serve with a tomato or cheese dip.

Nutrition Information: Calories 83; Total Fat 3g; Sodium 173mg; Total Carbs 4g; Net Carbs 4g; Protein 3g

Tasty Carrot Crisps

[Prep + Cook Time: 20 Minutes | **Serves:** 2]

Ingredients:

- 3 large Carrots, washed and peeled
- Salt to season
- Olive Oil Cooking Spray

Directions:

1. Using a mandolin slicer, slice the carrots very thinly height wise. Put the carrot strips in a bowl and season with salt to taste
2. Open the Air Fryer, grease the fryer basket lightly with cooking spray, and add the carrot strips to it. Close the Air Fryer and fry at 350°F for 6 minutes
3. Pull out the fryer basket, and stir the carrots with a spoon. Cook further for 4 minutes or until crispy. Serve with dipping sauce of your choice

Nutrition Information: Calories 35; Total Fat 0g; Sodium 65mg; Total Carbs 8g; Net Carbs 6g; Protein 1g

Zucchini Chips

[Prep + Cook Time: 1 hour 10 Minutes | **Serves:** 3 to 4]

Ingredients:

- 1 cup Keto Breadcrumbs
- 3 medium Zucchinis
- 1 teaspoon Smoked Paprika
- 2 Eggs, beaten
- 1 cup grated Parmesan Cheese
- Salt and Pepper to taste
- Cooking Spray

Directions:

1. With a mandolin cutter, slice the zucchinis thinly. Use paper towels to press out excess liquid
2. In a bowl, add the breadcrumbs, salt, pepper, cheese, and paprika. Mix well and set aside. Place a wire rack or tray aside.
3. Now, dip each zucchini slice in egg and then in the cheese mix while pressing to coat them well in cheese. Place them on the wire rack.
4. Spray the coated slices with cooking spray. Open the Air Fryer, place the slices in the fryer basket in a single layer without overlapping.
5. Close the Air Fryer and cook them at 350°F for 8 minutes for each batch
6. Once ready, remove them onto a serving platter and sprinkle with salt. Serve with spicy dip

Nutrition Information: Calories 140; Total Fat 9g; Sodium 280mg; Total Carbs 1g; Net Carbs 1g; Protein 4g

Mixed Sweet Nuts

[**Prep + Cook Time:** 25 Minutes | **Serves:** 5]

Ingredients:
- 1/2 cup Walnuts
- 1/2 cup Almonds
- 1/2 cup Pecans
- 2 tablespoon Egg Whites
- 2 teaspoon Cinnamon
- 2 tablespoon Stevia Sweetener
- A pinch Ground Cayenne
- Cooking Spray

Directions:
1. Preheat Air Fryer to 300°F. Add the pepper, stevia, and cinnamon to a bowl and mix them well. Set aside.
2. In another bowl, pour in the pecans, walnuts, almonds, and egg whites. Mix well
3. Add the spice mixture to the nuts and give it a good mix.
4. Open the Air Fryer and lightly grease the fryer basket with cooking spray
5. Pour in the nuts, close the Air Fryer, and bake them for 10 minutes.
6. Open the Air Fryer, stir the nuts using a wooden vessel, close the Air Fryer, and bake further for 10 minutes.
7. Set a bowl ready and once the timer is done, pour the nuts in the bowl. Let cool before crunching on them as they are

Nutrition Information: Calories 170; Total Fat 15g; Sodium 85mg; Total Carbs 5g; Net Carbs 3g; Protein 6g

Tortilla Chips

[**Prep + Cook Time:** 55 Minutes | **Serves:** 3]

Ingredients:
- 1 cup Almond Flour
- 2 cups shredded Cheddar Cheese
- 1 tablespoon Golden Flaxseed Meal
- Salt and Pepper to taste
- Cooking Spray

Directions:
1. Preheat the Air Fryer to 350°F. Pour the cheddar cheese in a medium sized microwave safe dish and melt it in the microwave for 1 minute. Remove the bowl in 15 second intervals to stir the cheese
2. Once melted, remove the bowl and quickly add the almond flour, salt, flaxseed meal, and pepper. Mix well with a fork.
3. On a chopping board, place the dough, and knead it with your hands while warm until the ingredients are well combined.
4. Divide the dough into two and using a rolling pin, roll them out flat into two rectangles.
5. Use a pastry cutter, to cut out triangle-shaped pieces and line them in 1 layer on a baking dish
6. Open the Air Fryer and grease the fryer basket lightly with cooking spray.
7. Arrange some triangle chips in 1 layer in the fryer basket without touching or overlapping. Spray them lightly with cooking spray. Close the Air Fryer and cook for 8 minutes. Serve with a cheese dip

Nutrition Information: Calories 165; Total Fat 14.4g; Sodium 117mg; Total Carbs 3.07g; Net Carbs 3.07g; Protein 4.57g

Mozzarella Sticks

[Prep + Cook Time: 2 hours 20 Minutes | **Serves:** 4]

Ingredients:

- 12 Mozzarella String Cheese
- 4 tablespoon Skimmed Milk
- 3 Eggs
- 2 cups Ground Pork Rinds

Directions:

1. Pour the pork rinds in a medium bowl. Crack the eggs into another bowl and beat with the milk
2. One after the other, dip each cheese sticks in the egg mixture, in the pork rinds, then egg mixture again and then in the pork rinds again.
3. Place the coated cheese sticks on a cookie sheet and freeze for 1 to 2 hours
4. Preheat the Air Fryer to 380°F.
5. Pull out the fryer basket and arrange the cheese sticks in it without overcrowding
6. Slide the fryer basket back in and cook for 5 minutes, flipping them halfway to brown evenly
7. Remove them to a plate and repeat the cooking process for the remaining sticks. Serve with a tomato dip

Nutrition Information: Calories 48; Total Fat 2g; Sodium 206mg; Total Carbs 0g; Net Carbs 0g; Protein 9g

Keto Onion Rings

[Prep + Cook Time: 20 Minutes | **Serves:** 2]

Ingredients:

- 1 large Onion, peeled and sliced into 1-inch rings
- 1 cup Almond Flour
- 2 medium Eggs, beaten
- 1 teaspoon Paprika Powder
- 3/4 cup Parmesan Cheese
- 1 teaspoon Garlic Powder
- A pinch of salt

Directions:

1. Preheat the Air Fryer to 350°F. Add the eggs to a bowl. Set aside. In another bowl, add the cheese, garlic powder, salt, almond flour, and paprika powder. Mix them using a spoon
2. Dip each onion ring in egg, then in the cheese mixture, in the egg again and finally in the cheese mixture.
3. Slide out the fryer basket and add the rings to it. Cook them for 8 minutes
4. Remove them onto a serving platter and serve with a cheese or tomatoes dip of choice

Nutrition Information: Calories 110; Total Fat 0g; Sodium 360mg; Total Carbs 1g; Net Carbs 1g; Protein 2g

Keto Sausage Balls

[Prep + Cook Time: 60 Minutes | **Serves:** 7]

Ingredients:

- 1½-pound Ground Sausages
- 2 ¼ cups Cheddar Cheese, shredded
- 3/4 cups Almond Flour
- 1/2 cup Coconut Flour
- 1 teaspoon Smoked Paprika
- 2 teaspoon Garlic Powder
- 1/2 cup melted Coconut Oil, leave to cool
- 3/4 cup Sour Cream
- 3/4 teaspoon Baking Soda
- 1 teaspoon dried Oregano
- 4 Eggs

Directions:

1. Place a pan over medium heat on a stove top, add the sausages and brown for 3 to 4 minutes. Drain the excess fat derived from cooking and set aside
2. Add the baking soda, almond flour, and coconut flour to a sifter and sift them into a bowl. Place aside.
3. In another bowl, add the eggs, sour cream, oregano, paprika, coconut oil, and garlic powder. Whisk to combine well

4. Combine the egg and flour mixtures using a spatula. Add the cheese and sausages. Fold in and let it sit for 5 minutes to thicken
5. Rub your hands with coconut oil and mold out bite-size balls out of the batter. Place them on a tray, and refrigerate for 15 minutes
6. Remove the sausage balls from the fridge, slide out the fryer basket, and add as much of the balls to it without overcrowding.
7. Slide the fryer basket in and cook them for 10 minutes per round
8. Transfer to a serving platter once ready and repeat the cooking process for any remaining balls. Serve with salsa

Nutrition Information: Calories 56; Total Fat 3.61g; Sodium 128mg; Total Carbs 0g; Net Carbs 0g; Protein 2.6g

Bacon Wrapped Avocados

[**Prep + Cook Time:** 40 Minutes | **Serves:** 6]

Ingredients:
- 12 thick strips Bacon
- 3 large and firm Avocados
- 1/3 teaspoon Cumin Powder
- 1/3 teaspoon Chili Powder
- 1/3 teaspoon Salt

Directions:
1. Using a knife, cut open the avocados, remove the seeds and slice them into 24 pieces without the skin. Set aside
2. Stretch the bacon strips to elongate them and use a knife to cut in half to make 24 pieces
3. Wrap each piece of bacon around each slice of avocado from one end to the other end. Tuck the end of bacon into the wrap.
4. Arrange the wrapped avocado on a flat surface and sprinkle with salt, chili and cumin powder on both sides.
5. Slide out the fryer basket and arrange 4 to 8 wrapped pieces in it
6. Slide the fryer basket in and cook at 350°F for 8 minutes or until the bacon is browned and crunchy, flipping half way through to cook evenly
7. Remove onto a wire rack and repeat the process for the remaining avocado pieces. Serve at room temperature

Nutrition Information: Calories 35; Total Fat 5g; Sodium 116mg; Total Carbs 10g; Net Carbs 10g; Protein 4g

Crusted Coconut Shrimp

[**Prep + Cook Time:** 30 Minutes | **Serves:** 5]

Ingredients:
- 1-pound Jumbo Shrimp, peeled and deveined
- 1/2 cup Keto Breadcrumbs
- 3/4 cup Shredded Coconut, unsweetened
- 1/3 cup Arrowroot Starch
- 1/2 cup Coconut Milk
- 1 tablespoon Monk Fruit Syrup

Directions:
1. Pour the arrowroot starch in a zipper bag, add the shrimp, zip the bag up and shake vigorously to coat the shrimp with the arrowroot starch
2. Preheat the Air Fryer to 350°F. Mix the monk fruit syrup and coconut milk in a bowl and place it aside.
3. In a separate bowl, mix the breadcrumbs and shredded coconut
4. Open the zipper bag and remove each shrimp while shaking off excess starch on it.
5. Dip each shrimp in the coconut milk mixture and then in the breadcrumbs mixture while pressing loosely to trap enough breadcrumbs and shredded coconut
6. Slide out the fryer basket and place the coated shrimp in it without overcrowding.
7. Close the Air Fryer and cook the shrimp for 6 to 8 minutes

8. Open the Air Fryer, flip the shrimp, and continue cooking for 3 to 4 minutes or until golden brown. Serve the shrimp with a coconut based dip

Nutrition Information: Calories 260; Total Fat 14g; Sodium 670mg; Total Carbs 6g; Net Carbs 2g; Protein 8g

Keto Radish Chips

[**Prep + Cook Time:** 35 Minutes | **Serves:** 4]

Ingredients:
- 10 Radishes, leaves removed and cleaned
- Cooking Spray
- Salt to season
- Water

Directions:
1. With a mandolin slicer, slice the radishes thinly. Place the radishes in a pot and pour in water to cover them up
2. Place the pot over medium heat on a stovetop and bring the water to boil until the radishes turn translucent about 4 minutes
3. After 4 minutes, drain the radishes through a sieve. Set aside.
4. Open the Air Fryer and grease the fryer basket with cooking spray
5. Add the radish slices into the fryer basket
6. Close the air fryer, and cook for 8 minutes or until they are a deep golden brown color.
7. Meanwhile, prepare a paper towel-lined plate
8. Once the radishes are ready, transfer them to the paper towel-lined plate. Season with salt and serve.

Nutrition Information: Calories 48; Total Fat 2.7g; Sodium 244mg; Total Carbs 2g; Net Carbs 0.2g; Protein 0.8g

Salami Sticks

[**Prep + Cook Time:** 2 hours 20 Minutes | **Serves:** 2]

Ingredients:
- 1-pound Ground Beef or Pork
- 1 teaspoon Liquid Smoke
- 3 tablespoon Monk Fruit Powder
- A pinch Garlic Powder
- A pinch Chili Powder
- Salt to taste

Directions:
1. Place the meat, monk fruit powder, garlic powder, chili powder, salt and liquid smoke in a bowl. Mix with a spoon
2. Mold out four sticks with your hands, place them on a plate, and refrigerate approximately for 2 hours
3. Preheat the Air Fryer to 350°F. Slide out the fryer basket and add the salami sticks to it. Cook for 10 minutes. Serve with a dipping sauce of choice

Nutrition Information: Calories 58; Total Fat 4.63g; Sodium 245mg; Total Carbs 0.52g; Net Carbs 0.52g; Protein 3.2g

Chicken Nuggets

[**Prep + Cook Time:** 1 hour 25 Minutes | **Serves:** 3]

Ingredients:
- 2 Chicken Breasts, all skin, fats, and bones removed
- 2 cups Almond Flour
- 2 cups Keto Breadcrumbs
- 2 tablespoon Paprika
- 4 teaspoon Onion Powder
- 1½ teaspoon Garlic Powder
- 2 cups of Milk
- Cooking Spray
- 2 Eggs
- Salt and Pepper to taste

Directions:
1. Cut the chicken into 1-inch chunks. In a small bowl, add the paprika, onion powder, garlic powder, salt, pepper, almond flour, and breadcrumbs. Mix well

2. In another bowl, crack the eggs, add the milk and beat them together
3. Prepare a tray aside. Dip each chicken chunk in the egg mixture, place them on the tray, and refrigerate for 1 hour. Preheat the Air Fryer to 370°F
4. After 1 hour, remove the chicken and roll each chunk in the breadcrumb mixture.
5. Open the Air Fryer and place the crusted chicken in the fryer basket. Spray with cooking spray. Slide in the fryer basket and cook for 4 minutes
6. Pull out the fryer basket, flip the chicken chunks, spray with cooking spray, and cook further for 4 minutes. Prepare a wire rack and remove the chicken onto it once ready
7. Serve the nuggets with a tomato dipping sauce or sugar-free ketchup. Yum!

Nutrition Information: Calories 48; Total Fat 3.01g; Sodium 92mg; Total Carbs 1g; Net Carbs 0.9g; Protein 2.49g

Keto Cheese Lings

[**Prep + Cook Time:** 25 Minutes | **Serves:** 3]

Ingredients:
- 1 cup Almond Flour + extra for kneading
- 1/2 teaspoon Baking Powder
- 3 teaspoon Butter
- 4 tablespoon grated Cheese + extra for rolling
- 1/4 teaspoon Chili Powder
- Water
- A pinch of Salt

Directions:
1. In a bowl, add the cheese, almond flour, baking powder, chili powder, butter, and salt. Mix well. The mixture should be crusty
2. Add some drops of water and mix well to get a dough. Remove the dough onto a chopping board or a flat surface
3. Rub some extra flour in your palms and knead the dough for a while
4. Sprinkle some more flour on the flat surface and using a rolling pin, roll the dough out into a thin sheet.
5. With a pastry cutter, cut the dough into your desired shapes.
6. Preheat the Air Fryer to 350°F. Pull out the fryer basket and add the cheese lings
7. Close the Air Fryer and cook for 2 minutes. Open the Air Fryer, toss the cheese lings, and continue cooking for 3 minutes

Nutrition Information: Calories 112; Total Fat 5.66g; Sodium 222mg; Total Carbs 3.55g; Net Carbs 3.15g; Protein 2.78g

Keto Egg Bread

[**Prep + Cook Time:** 12 Minutes | **Serves:** 2]

Ingredients:
- 2 slices Keto Bread
- 2 Eggs
- 2 tablespoon Butter
- Salt and Pepper to taste

Directions:
1. Place a 3 X 3 cm heatproof bowl in the fryer basket and brush with butter
2. Make a hole in the middle of the bread slices with a bread knife and place in the heatproof bowl in 2 batches.
3. Break an egg into the center of each hole. Season with salt and pepper
4. Close the Air Fryer and cook for 4 minutes at 330°F
5. Turn the bread with a spatula and cook for another 4 minutes. Serve as a breakfast accompaniment

Nutrition Information: Calories: 220; Total Fat: 16g; Sodium: 459mg; Total Carbs: 10g; Net Carbs: 1g; Protein: 8g

Keto Chicken Wingettes

[Prep + Cook Time: 45 Minutes | **Serves:** 3]

Ingredients:
- 15 Chicken Wingettes
- 1/3 cup Butter
- 1/2 tablespoon White Vinegar
- 1/3 cup Hot Sauce
- Salt and Pepper to taste

Directions:
1. Preheat the Air Fryer to 360°F. Season the wingettes with pepper and salt
2. Slide out the fryer basket, add the wingettes to it and cook for 35 minutes. Toss them every 5 minutes
3. Once read, remove them into a bowl. Over low heat on a stove top, place a saucepan, add the butter and melt it.
4. Add the vinegar and hot sauce. Stir and cook for a minute. Turn the heat off
5. Pour the sauce over the chicken. Toss to coat well.
6. Transfer the chicken to a serving platter. Serve with a side of celery strips and blue cheese dressing

Nutrition Information: Calories 563; Total Fat 28g; Sodium 774mg; Total Carbs 2g; Net Carbs 1.8g; Protein 35g

Salmon Croquettes

[Prep + Cook Time: 40 Minutes | **Serves:** 3]

Ingredients:
- 3 (15 oz) Tinned Salmon, deboned and flaked
- 1½ cups grated Carrots
- 1 cup grated Onion
- 2½ teaspoon Italian Seasoning
- 2½ teaspoon Lemon Juice
- 4 tablespoon Mayonnaise
- 3 large Eggs
- 1½ tablespoon chopped Chives
- 4 tablespoon Keto Breadcrumbs
- Cooking Spray
- Salt and Pepper to taste

Directions:
1. In a mixing bowl, add the salmon, onion, carrots, eggs, chives, mayonnaise, breadcrumbs, Italian seasoning, pepper, salt, and lemon juice and mix well
2. Using your hands, form 2-inch thick oblong balls from the mixture of as much as you can get
3. Put the croquettes on a flat tray and refrigerate for 45 minutes to make compact.
4. Pull out the fryer basket and grease with cooking spray. Remove the croquettes from the fridge and in a single layer, arrange in the fryer basket without overcrowding. Re-spray them with cooking spray
5. Slide the fryer basket in and cook for 6 minutes until crispy.
6. Open the Air Fryer, flip the patties, spray with oil, and continue cooking for 4 minutes
7. Once ready, transfer the croquettes to a serving platter and serve warm with a dill based dip

Nutrition Information: Calories 166; Total Fat 10g; Sodium 72mg; Total Carbs 1g; Net Carbs 1g; Protein 28.52g

Vegan & Vegetarian

Curried Cauliflower Florets

[Prep + Cook Time: 35 Minutes | **Serves:** 4]

Ingredients:
- 1 large Cauliflower Head
- 1½ tablespoon Curry Powder
- 1/2 cup Olive Oil
- 1/3 cup Fried Pine Nuts
- Salt to taste

Directions:
1. Preheat the Air Fryer to 390°F. Add the pine nuts and 1 teaspoon of olive oil in a medium bowl. Mix with the tablespoon
2. Pour them in the fryer basket and cook them for 2 minutes. Remove them into a bowl to cool. Place the cauliflower on a cutting board
3. Use a knife to cut them it into 1-inch florets. Place them in a large mixing bowl
4. Add the curry powder, salt, and the remaining olive oil and mix well
5. Place the cauliflower florets in the fryer basket in 2 batches and cook each batch for 10 minutes.
6. Remove the curried florets onto a serving platter, sprinkle with the pine nuts, and toss. Serve the florets with a tomato sauce or a side to a meat dish

Nutrition Information: Calories: 140; Total Fat: 3g; Sodium: 370mg; Total Carbs: 0g; Net Carbs: 0g; Protein: 5g

Brussels Sprouts with Garlic

[Prep + Cook Time: 25 Minutes | **Serves:** 4]

Ingredients:
- 1-pound Brussels Sprouts, trimmed and excess leaves removed
- 3 cloves Garlic
- 3/4 cup Mayonnaise, whole egg
- 2 cups Water
- 2 teaspoon Lemon Juice
- 1 teaspoon Powdered Chili
- 1½ tablespoon Olive Oil
- Salt and Pepper to taste

Directions:
1. Place a skillet over medium heat on a stove top, add the garlic cloves with the peels on it and roast until lightly brown and fragrant
2. Remove the skillet with the garlic and place a pot with water over the same heat. Bring it to a boil.
3. Using a knife, cut the Brussels sprouts in halves lengthwise. Add to the boiling water to blanch for just 3 minutes. Drain through a sieve and set aside.
4. Preheat the Air Fryer to 350°F. Remove the garlic from the skillet to a plate; peel and crush and set aside.
5. Add olive oil to the skillet and light the fire to medium heat on the stove top
6. Stir in the Brussels sprouts, season with pepper and salt. Sauté for 2 minutes. Turn off the heat.
7. Pour the Brussels sprouts in the fryer basket and bake for 5 minutes
8. Meanwhile, make the garlic aioli. In a bowl, add the mayonnaise, crushed garlic, lemon juice, powdered chili, pepper and salt in a bowl. Mix well
9. Remove the Brussels sprouts onto a serving bowl and serve with the garlic aioli

Nutrition Information: Calories: 42; Total Fat: 2.26g; Sodium: 342mg; Total Carbs: 0g; Net Carbs: 0g; Protein: 4.97g

Double Cheese Vegetable Frittata

[Prep + Cook Time: 35 Minutes | **Serves:** 2]

Ingredients:

- 1/4-pound Asparagus, trimmed and sliced thinly
- 1 cup Baby Spinach
- 1 small Red Onion, sliced
- 1/4 cup chopped Chives
- 2 teaspoon Olive Oil
- 4 Eggs, cracked into a bowl
- 1/3 cup Sliced Mushrooms
- 1/3 cup grated Cheddar Cheese
- 1/3 cup crumbled Feta Cheese
- 1 large Zucchini, sliced with a 1-inch thickness
- 1/3 cup Milk
- Salt and Pepper to taste

Directions:

1. Preheat the Air Fryer to 320°F. Line a 3 X 3 baking dish with parchment paper. Set aside
2. In the egg bowl, add the milk, salt, and pepper. Beat evenly.
3. Place a skillet over medium heat on a stove top, add olive oil.
4. Once heated, add the asparagus, zucchini, onion, mushrooms, and baby spinach
5. Sauté for 5 minutes while stirring. Pour the sautéed veggies into the baking dish and pour the egg mixture over.
6. Sprinkle the feta and cheddar cheese over it and place it in the Air Fryer
7. Close the Air Fryer and cook it for 15 minutes
8. Once ready, remove the baking dish and garnish with the fresh chives. Serve the frittata slices as they are.

Nutrition Information: Calories: 203; Total Fat: 10.23g; Sodium: 323mg; Total Carbs: 0g; Net Carbs: 0g; Protein: 6.41g

Cheesy Mushroom, Cauliflower Balls

[Prep + Cook Time: 50 Minutes | **Serves:** 5]

Ingredients:

- 1/2-pound Mushrooms, diced
- 1 small Red Onion, chopped
- 1 cup Grana Padano
- 1/4 cup Coconut Oil
- 3 tablespoon Olive Oil
- 3 cups Cauli Rice
- 3 cloves garlic, minced
- 2 sprigs Chopped Fresh Thyme
- 1 cup Keto Breadcrumbs
- 2 tablespoon Chicken Stock
- Salt and Pepper to taste

Directions:

1. Place a skillet over medium heat on a stove top. Add olive oil, once heated add the garlic and onion. Sauté until translucent
2. Add the mushrooms, stir and cook for about 4 minutes. Add the cauli rice and constantly stir-fry for 5 minutes
3. Add the chicken stock, thyme, and simmer until the cauli rice has absorbed the stock.
4. Add Grana Padano cheese, pepper, and salt. Stir and turn off the heat.
5. Allow the mixture cool and make bite-size balls of the mixture. Place them in a plate and refrigerate them for 30 minutes to harden
6. Preheat the Air Fryer to 350°F. In a bowl, add the keto breadcrumbs and coconut oil and mix well.
7. Remove the mushroom balls from the refrigerator, stir the breadcrumb mixture again, and roll the balls in the breadcrumb mixture
8. Place the balls in the fryer basket without overcrowding and cook for 15 minutes while tossing every 5 minutes for an even cook
9. Repeat this process until all the mushroom balls have fried. Serve them with sautéed zoodles and tomato sauce

Nutrition Information: Calories: 95; Total Fat: 5.68g; Sodium: 85mg; Total Carbs: 4.12g; Net Carbs: 3g; Protein: 5.76g

Vegetable Croquettes

[**Prep + Cook Time:** 1 hour 35 Minutes | **Serves:** 4]

Ingredients:

- 1-pound Turnips
- 2 Red Peppers, chopped
- 1/2 cup Baby Spinach, chopped
- 3 Mushrooms, chopped
- 1/2 Red Onion, chopped
- 2 cloves Garlic, minced
- 1 medium Carrot, grated
- 2 cups Water
- 2 teaspoon Olive Oil
- 1/3 cup Almond Flour
- 1 cup Unsweetened Almond Milk
- 1/4 cup Coconut Milk
- 1/6 Broccoli Florets, chopped
- 1/6 cup sliced Green Onion
- 2 teaspoon + 3 teaspoon Vegan Butter
- 2 tablespoon Arrowroot Starch
- 1½ cups Keto Breadcrumbs
- Olive Oil Cooking Spray
- Salt to taste

Directions:

1. Place the turnips in a pot, add the water, and bring it to boil over medium heat on a stove top. Boil until tender and mashable
2. Drain the turnips through a sieve and pour them into a bowl. Add the 2 teaspoons of vegan butter, coconut milk, and salt. Use a potato masher to mash well and set aside
3. Place a skillet over medium heat on a stove top and add the remaining vegan butter. Once it melts, add the onion, garlic, red peppers, broccoli, and mushrooms. Stir and cook the veggies for 2 minutes.
4. Add the green onion and spinach. Cook until the spinach wilts
5. Season with a bit of salt and stir. Turn the heat off and pour the veggie mixture in the turnip mash.
6. Use the potato masher to mash the veggies into the turnip. Allow cooling.
7. Using your hands, form oblong balls of the mixture and place them on a baking sheet in a single layer.
8. Refrigerate them for 30 minutes. In 3 separate bowls, pour the keto breadcrumbs in one, almond flour in the second bowl, and cornstarch, almond milk and salt in the third bowl
9. Mix the cornstarch with the almond milk and salt with a fork. Remove the patties from the fridge. Preheat the Air Fryer to 390°F
10. Dredge each veggie mold in almond flour, then in the cornstarch mixture, and then in the breadcrumbs. Place the patties in batches in a single layer in the fryer basket without overlapping
11. Spray them with olive oil cooking spray and cook them for 2 minutes
12. Flip and spray them with cooking spray and continue cooking for 3 minutes. Remove them onto a wire rack and serve with tomato sauce

Nutrition Information: Calories: 24; Total Fat: 0.23g; Sodium: 20mg; Total Carbs: 2.46g; Net Carbs: 0.76g; Protein: 3.13g

Hash Browns

[**Prep + Cook Time:** 1 hour 25 Minutes | **Serves:** 3]

Ingredients:
- 7 Radishes, peeled
- 1 Egg, beaten
- 1 teaspoon Chili Flakes
- 1 teaspoon Onion Powder
- 1 tablespoon Olive Oil
- 1 teaspoon Garlic Powder
- Cooking Spray
- Salt and Pepper to taste

Directions:
1. Using a shredder, shred the radishes and place them in cheesecloth. Squeeze in the cloth to extract the extra moisture in them
2. Place a skillet over medium heat on a stove top, add the olive oil and radishes. Sauté until turn evenly golden, about 20 to 30 minutes.
3. Transfer the radishes into a bowl and let them cool completely
4. After they have cooled, add in the egg, pepper, salt, chili flakes, onion powder, and garlic powder. Mix well.
5. In a flat plate, spread the mixture and pat firmly with your fingers
6. Refrigerate for 20 minutes and preheat the Air Fryer to 350°F. Remove from the fridge and use a knife to divide it into equal sizes.
7. Grease the fryer basket of the Air Fryer with cooking spray and place the patties in the basket.
8. Close the Air Fryer and cook them at 350°F for 15 minutes
9. Open the Air Fryer and turn the hash browns with a spatula. Cook further for 6 minutes. Serve with sunshine eggs

Nutrition Information: Calories: 312; Total Fat: 15g; Sodium: 808mg; Total Carbs: 4g; Net Carbs: 1.6g; Protein: 16g

Cheesy Broccoli Quiche

[**Prep + Cook Time:** 50 Minutes | **Serves:** 2]

Ingredients:
- 2 medium Broccoli, cut into florets
- 2 medium Tomatoes, diced
- 1 teaspoon dried Thyme
- 1/4 cup Feta Cheese, crumbled
- 1 cup grated Cheddar Cheese
- 4 Eggs
- 4 medium Carrots, diced
- 1 teaspoon chopped Parsley
- 1 cup Whole Milk
- Salt and Pepper to taste

Directions:
1. Put the broccoli and carrots in a food steamer and cook until soft, about 10 minutes
2. In a jug, crack in the eggs, add the parsley, salt, pepper, and thyme. Using a whisk, beat the eggs while adding the milk gradually until a pale mixture is attained
3. Once the broccoli and carrots are ready, strain them through a sieve and set aside
4. In a 3 X 3 cm quiche dish, add the carrots and broccoli. Put the tomatoes on top, then the feta and cheddar cheese following. Leave a little cheddar cheese.
5. Pour the egg mixture over the layering and top with the remaining cheddar cheese
6. Place the dish in the Air Fryer and cook at 350°F for 20 minutes. Once ready, remove the dish, use a knife to cut out slices, and serve

Nutrition Information: Calories: 316; Total Fat: 23.89g; Sodium: 292mg; Total Carbs: 0g; Net Carbs: 0g; Protein: 9.91g

Italian Tofu

[Prep + Cook Time: 30 Minutes | **Serves:** 2]

Ingredients:

- 6-ounce extra firm Tofu
- 1 tablespoon Sugar-free Soy Sauce
- 1/3 teaspoon Onion Powder
- 1/3 teaspoon Garlic Powder
- 1/3 teaspoon dried Basil
- 1 tablespoon Vegetable Broth
- 1/3 teaspoon dried Oregano
- Pepper to season

Directions:

1. Place the tofu on a cutting board. Cut it into 3 lengthwise slices with a knife
2. Line a side of the cutting board with paper towels, place the tofu on it and cover with paper towel.
3. Use your hands to press the tofu gently until as much liquid has been extracted from it
4. Remove the paper towels and use a knife to chop the tofu into 8 cubes. Put them in a bowl and set aside
5. In another bowl, add the soy sauce, vegetable broth, oregano, basil, garlic powder, onion powder, and black pepper. Mix well with a spoon
6. Pour the spice mixture on the tofu, stir the tofu until well coated, and place it aside to marinate for 10 minutes. Preheat the Air Fryer to 390°F
7. Arrange the tofu in the fryer basket in a single layer. Cook the tofu for 6 minutes.
8. Slide out the fryer basket and turn the tofu using a spatula
9. Slide it back in and continue cooking for 4 minutes. Remove them onto a plate and serve with a side of green salad

Nutrition Information: Calories: 87; Total Fat: 4.4g; Sodium: 452mg; Total Carbs: 3.4g; Net Carbs: 2.3g; Protein: 10g

Eggplant Gratin with Crispy Mozzarella Crust

[Prep + Cook Time: 30 Minutes | **Serves:** 2]

Ingredients:

- 1 cup cubed Eggplant
- 1/4 cup chopped Yellow Onion
- 1/3 cup chopped Tomatoes
- 1/4 cup grated Mozzarella Cheese
- 1 teaspoon Capers
- 1/4 teaspoon dried Basil
- 1/4 teaspoon dried Marjoram
- 1/4 cup chopped Red Pepper
- 1/4 cup chopped Green Pepper
- 1 clove Garlic, minced
- 1 tablespoon sliced Pimiento Stuffed Olives
- 1 tablespoon Keto Breadcrumbs
- Olive Oil Cooking Spray
- Salt and Pepper to taste

Directions:

1. Preheat the Air Fryer to 300°F. In a bowl, add the eggplant, green pepper, red pepper, onion, tomatoes, olives, garlic, basil marjoram, capers, salt, and pepper
2. Lightly grease a 3 X 3 baking dish with the olive oil cooking spray. Ladle the eggplant mixture into the baking dish and level it using the vessel
3. Sprinkle the mozzarella cheese on top of it and top it with the keto breadcrumbs. Place the dish in the Air Fryer and cook it for 20 minutes. Serve with cauli rice

Nutrition Information: Calories: 317; Total Fat: 16.83g; Sodium: 655mg; Total Carbs: 2g; Net Carbs: 2g; Protein: 12g

Stuffed Garlic Mushrooms

[Prep + Cook Time: 20 Minutes | **Serves:** 3]

Ingredients:

- 14 small Button Mushrooms
- 1 tablespoon chopped Parsley
- 1 clove Garlic, minced
- 4 slices Bacon, chopped
- 1/4 cup grated Cheddar Cheese
- 1 tablespoon Olive Oil
- salt and Pepper to taste

Directions:

1. Preheat the Air Fryer to 390°F. In a bowl, add the olive oil, bacon, cheddar cheese, parsley, salt, pepper, and garlic. Mix them well using a spoon
2. Cut the stalks of the mushroom off and fill each cap with the bacon mixture
3. Press the bacon mixture into the caps to avoid any from falling off.
4. Place the stuffed mushrooms in the fryer basket, close the Air Fryer and cook at 390°F for 8 minutes
5. Once golden and crispy, remove them onto a serving platter. Serve with a green leaf salad

Nutrition Information: Calories: 67; Total Fat: 3.51g; Sodium: 142mg; Total Carbs: 0.12g; Net Carbs: 0.9g; Protein: 2.77g

Eggplant, Parsnips, and Zucchini Chips

[Prep + Cook Time: 50 Minutes | **Serves:** 4]

Ingredients:

- 1 large Eggplant
- 3 medium Zucchinis
- 1/2 cup Olive Oil
- 1/2 cup Arrowroot Starch
- 5 medium Parsnips
- 1/2 cup Water
- Salt to season

Directions:

1. Preheat the Air Fryer to 390°F. Cut the eggplant and zucchini in long 3-inch strips. Peel the parsnips and cut them in 3-inch strips. Place aside
2. In a bowl, add the arrowroot starch, water, salt, pepper, olive oil, eggplants, zucchini, and parsnips and sir well to combine
3. Place one-third of the veggie strips in the fryer basket, close the Air Fryer and cook them for 12 minutes. Once ready, transfer them to a serving platter
4. Repeat the cooking process for the remaining veggie strips until they are all done. Serve warm as a side to a meat dish or with spicy or sweet sauce

Nutrition Information:

Calories: 120; Total Fat: 3.5g; Sodium: 240mg; Total Carbs: 6g; Net Carbs: 6g; Protein: 3g

Keto Tomato Sandwiches with Feta and Pesto

[Prep + Cook Time: 60 Minutes | **Serves:** 2]

Ingredients:

- 1 Heirloom Tomato
- 1 (4- oz.) block Feta Cheese
- 1/4 cup chopped Parsley
- 1 clove Garlic
- 2 teaspoon + 1/4 cup Olive Oil
- 1½ tbsp. Toasted Pine Nuts
- 1/4 cup grated Parmesan Cheese
- 1/4 cup chopped Basil
- 1 small Red Onion, thinly sliced
- Salt to taste

Directions:

1. Start with the pesto: Add the basil, pine nuts, garlic and salt to the food processor. Process it while adding the 1/4 cup of olive oil slowly
2. Once the oil is finished, pour the basil pesto into a bowl and refrigerate it for 30 minutes
3. Preheat the Air Fryer to 390°F. Slice the feta cheese and tomato into ½ inch circular slices

4. Use a kitchen towel to pat the tomatoes dry. Remove the pesto from the fridge and use a tablespoon to spread some pesto on each slice of tomato. Top with a slice of feta cheese
5. Add the onion and remaining olive oil in a bowl and toss. Spoon on top of the feta cheese on the tomato.
6. Carefully place the tomato in the fryer basket, close the air fryer, and bake it for 12 minutes
7. Remove the tomatoes onto a serving platter, sprinkle lightly with salt and top with any remaining pesto. Serve with a side of cauli rice

Nutrition Information: Calories: 41; Total Fat: 4g; Sodium: 25mg; Total Carbs: 5g; Net Carbs: 3g; Protein: 2g

Roast Winter Vegetable Delight

[Prep + Cook Time: 30 Minutes | **Serves:** 2]

Ingredients:

- 1 small Parsnip, peeled and sliced in a 2-inch thickness
- 1 cup chopped Celery
- 1 tablespoon chopped Fresh Thyme
- 1 cup chopped Butternut Squash
- 2 teaspoon Olive Oil
- 2 small Red Onions, cut in wedges
- Salt and Pepper to taste

Directions:

1. Preheat the Air Fryer to 200°F. In a bowl, add the parsnips, butternut squash, red onions, celery, thyme, pepper, salt, and olive oil and mix well
2. Pour the vegetables into the fryer basket, close the Air Fryer, and cook for 16 minutes. Transfer the roasted veggies into a serving bowl

Nutrition Information: Calories: 50; Total Fat: 3g; Sodium: 30mg; Total Carbs: 5g; Net Carbs: 3g; Protein: 2g

Keto Veg Bake

[Prep + Cook Time: 30 Minutes | **Serves:** 3]

Ingredients:

- 3 Turnips, sliced
- 2 cloves Garlic, crushed
- 1 Bay Leaf, cut in 6 pieces
- 1 tablespoon Olive Oil
- 1 large Zucchini, sliced
- 1 large Red Onion, cut into rings
- Salt and Pepper to season
- Cooking Spray

Directions:

1. Place the turnips, onion, and zucchini in a bowl. toss with olive oil and season with salt and pepper
2. Preheat the Air Fryer to 330°F. Place the veggies into a baking pan that fits in the Air Fryer.
3. Slip the bay leaves in the different parts of the slices and tuck the garlic cloves in between the slices
4. Insert the pan in the Air Fryer basket and cook for 15 minutes
5. Once ready, remove and serve warm with as a side to a meat dish or salad

Nutrition Information: Calories: 50; Total Fat: 2g; Sodium: 30mg; Total Carbs: 4g; Net Carbs: 2g; Protein: 2g

Cheesy Stuffed Peppers with Cauli Rice

[Prep + Cook Time: 40 Minutes | **Serves:** 4]

Ingredients:

- 4 Green Peppers, you can use any color of your choice
- 1 Red Onion, chopped
- 2 tablespoon chopped Basil
- 1 tablespoon Lemon Zest
- 1/2 cup Olive Oil
- 1 large Tomato, chopped
- 2 tablespoon grated Parmesan Cheese
- 1/2 cup crumbled Goat Cheese
- 3 cups Cauli Rice
- Salt and Pepper to taste

Directions:

1. Preheat the Air Fryer to 350°F. Cut the Peppers a quarter way from the head down and lengthwise. Remove the membrane and seeds
2. Season the Peppers with pepper, salt, and drizzle olive oil over

3. Place the Pepper bottoms in the fryer basket and cook them for 5 minutes at 350°F to soften them a little.
4. In a mixing bowl, add the tomatoes, goat cheese, lemon zest, basil, and cauli rice. Season with salt and pepper. Mix well
5. Remove the Pepper bottoms from the Air Fryer onto a flat surface and spoon the cheese mixture into them.
6. Sprinkle parmesan cheese on top of each and gently place in the fryer basket. Bake them for 15 minutes. Remove them once ready onto a serving platter

Nutrition Information: Calories: 115; Total Fat: 16g; Sodium: 300mg; Total Carbs: 0g; Net Carbs: 0g; Protein: 13g

Spicy Veggie Bites

[**Prep + Cook Time:** 2 hours 5 Minutes | **Serves:** 14 to 16]

Ingredients:
- 1 medium Cauliflower, cut in florets
- 2 Leeks, sliced thinly
- 1/2 cup Cauli Rice, not steamed
- 1 Onion, diced
- 1/2 cup Garden Peas
- 1 tablespoon Curry Paste
- 2 teaspoon Mixed Spice
- 1 teaspoon Ginger Paste
- 1 teaspoon Coriander
- 1 teaspoon Cumin Powder
- 1/3 cup Almond Flour
- 1 small Courgette, chopped
- 6 medium Carrots, diced
- 1 medium Broccoli, cut in florets
- 1 tablespoon Garlic Paste
- 2 tablespoon Olive Oil
- 1½ cups Coconut Milk
- Salt and Pepper to taste

Directions:
1. Steam all the vegetables except the leek and courgette for 10 minutes. Set aside
2. Place a wok over medium heat; add the onion, ginger, garlic and olive oil. Stir-fry until onions turn transparent. Add the leek, courgette and curry paste. Stir and cook for 5 minutes
3. Add all the listed spices, coconut milk, and cauli rice. Stir and simmer for 10 minutes
4. Once the sauce has reduced, add the steamed veggies. Mix evenly. Transfer into a bowl and refrigerate for 1 hour. Remove the veggie base from the fridge and mold into bite sizes.
5. Arrange the veggie bites in the fryer basket and close the Air Fryer. Cook at 350°F for 10 minutes
6. Once they are ready, it is time to serve them. Serve with yogurt dipping sauce for the best taste

Nutrition Information: Calories: 160; Total Fat: 8g; Sodium: 290mg; Total Carbs: 3g; Net Carbs: 2g; Protein: 3g

Roasted Rosemary Squash

[**Prep + Cook Time:** 30 Minutes | **Serves:** 2]

Ingredients:
- 1 Butternut Squash
- 1 tablespoon dried Rosemary
- Cooking Spray
- Salt to season

Directions:
1. Place the butternut squash on a cutting board and peel it. Cut it in half and remove the seeds. Cut the pulp into wedges and season with salt. Preheat the Air Fryer to 350°F. Spray the squash wedges with cooking spray and sprinkle the rosemary on it
2. Grease the fryer basket with cooking spray and place the wedges in it without overlapping. Slide the fryer basket back in and cook for 10 minutes
3. Flip the wedges and cook further for 10 minutes. Serve right away with a dip

Nutrition Information: Calories: 18; Total Fat: 0.2g; Sodium: 20mg; Total Carbs: 3.76g; Net Carbs: 2.56g; Protein: 1.3g

Desserts

Chocolate and Pecan Cupcakes

[Prep + Cook Time: 25 Minutes | **Serves:** 12]

Ingredients:
- 1/2 cup almond flour
- 1/2 teaspoon baking powder
- 2 tablespoons evaporated milk
- 1/4 teaspoon cardamom
- 1/4 teaspoon grated nutmeg
- 1 stick butter, at room temperature
- 1/3 cup swerve
- 2 tablespoons pecans, chopped
- 2-ounces low-carb chocolate chips

Directions:
1. Preheat your Air Fryer to 320 degrees F. Grease a muffin tin with a nonstick cooking spray
2. In a mixing bowl, sift the almond flour and baking powder
3. In another bowl, thoroughly combine the milk with butter, swerve, cardamom, and nutmeg. Fold in the chopped pecans and chocolate chips
4. Divide the mixture among muffin cups and transfer to your Air Fryer. Bake for 12 minutes
5. Turn off your Air Fryer and let the cupcakes sit for 8 minutes. Unmold your cupcakes and transfer them to a dessert platter. Serve and enjoy!

Nutrition Information: 132 Calories; 10.8g Fat; 8.8g Carbs; 1.3g Protein; 4.1g Sugars

Sunday Berry Cobbler

[Prep + Cook Time: 20 Minutes | **Serves:** 2]

Ingredients
- 1 cups mixed berries
- 1/4 cup swerve
- 2 tablespoons butter, melted
- 1/3 cup almond flour
- 2 tablespoons coconut oil, room temperature
- 1/4 teaspoon grated nutmeg
- 1/2 teaspoon ground cinnamon
- 1/3 teaspoon ground star anise
- A pinch of coarse salt

Directions
1. Start by preheating your Air Fryer to 360 degrees F for 5 minutes
2. Toss apple slices with swerve, butter, nutmeg, cinnamon, star anise, and salt. Top with almond flour mixed with coconut oil
3. Cook for 14 minutes, shaking halfway through cooking time. Store in an airtight container and enjoy!

Nutrition Information: 326 Calories; 32.5g Fat; 8.5g Carbs; 3.6g Protein; 2.6g Sugars

Lemon Curd

[Prep + Cook Time: 35 Minutes | **Serves:** 2]

Ingredients:
- 1 Egg Yolk
- 3 tablespoon Swerve Sugar
- 3/4 Lemon, juiced
- 3 tablespoon Butter
- 1 Egg

Directions:
1. Add the sugar and butter in a medium ramekin and use a hand mixer to beat evenly
2. Add the egg and yolk slowly while still whisking. Fresh yellow color will be attained
3. Add the lemon juice and mix it. Place the bowl in the fryer basket and start cooking at 170°F for 3 minutes. Then, increase the temperature to 190°F and cook for 3 minutes
4. Increase the temperature again to 210°F and cook for 6 minutes, then 230°F for 6 minutes, and finally to 250°F for 6 minutes.

5. Remove the bowl onto a flat surface. Use a spoon to check for any lumps and remove
6. Cover the ramekin with a plastic wrap and refrigerate it overnight or serve immediately

Nutrition Information: Calories: 60; Total Fat: 6g; Sodium: 50mg; Total Carbs: 0g; Net Carbs: 0g; Protein: 2g

Grandma's Butter Rum Cookies

[**Prep + Cook Time:** 25 Minutes | **Serves:** 10]

Ingredients:
- 1 cup almond flour
- 1 cup coconut flour
- 1 packet baking powder
- 1 cup swerve
- 2 tablespoons buttermilk
- 2 tablespoons rum
- 1/2 teaspoon sea salt
- 1 stick butter, at room temperature
- 1/2 teaspoon butter rum flavoring
- 2-ounces walnuts, finely chopped

Directions:
1. Begin by preheating the Air Fryer to 360 degrees F for 5 to 10 minutes
2. In a mixing dish, thoroughly combine the flour with baking powder and sea salt
3. Beat the butter and swerve with a hand mixer until pale and fluffy. Now, stir in the flour mixture
4. Add the remaining ingredients; mix to combine well. Divide the mixture into 14 small balls; flatten each ball with a fork and transfer them to a foil-lined baking pan
5. Put the baking pan into the Air Fryer and bake your cookies for 14 minutes. Work in a few batches, without crowding. Serve and enjoy!

Nutrition Information: 211 Calories; 20.5g Fat; 4.2g Carbs; 3.3g Protein; 1.2g Sugars

Chocolate and Butter Fondants

[**Prep + Cook Time:** 25 Minutes | **Serves:** 4]

Ingredients:
- 3/4 cup Dark Chocolate
- 1/4 cup + 1/4 cup Swerve Sugar
- 4 Eggs, room temperature
- 1/2 cup Peanut Butter, crunchy
- 2 tablespoon Butter, diced
- 1/8 cup Almond Flour, sieved
- 1/4 cup Water
- Cooking Spray
- 1 teaspoon Salt

Directions:
1. Make a salted praline to top the chocolate fondant. Add 1/4 cup of sugar, 1 teaspoon of salt and the water into a saucepan. Stir and bring it to a boil over low heat on a stove top. Simmer until the desired color is achieved and reduced
2. Pour it into a baking tray and leave it to cool and harden.
3. Preheat the Air Fryer to 300°F. Place a pot of water over medium heat and place a heatproof bowl over it
4. Add the chocolate, butter, and peanut butter to the bowl. Stir continuously until fully melted, combined, and smooth.
5. Remove the bowl from the heat and allow it to cool slightly.
6. Add the eggs to the chocolate and whisk it. Add the flour and remaining sugar and mix well
7. Grease 4 small loaf pans with cooking spray and divide the chocolate mixture between them.
8. Place the pans, 2 pans at a time in the fryer basket and bake for 7 minutes. Remove them and serve the fondants with a piece each salted praline

Nutrition Information: Calories: 157; Total Fat: 4g; Sodium: 11mg; Total Carbs: 4g; Net Carbs: 3.1g; Protein: 0.95g

The Ultimate Chocolate & Almond Muffins

[Prep + Cook Time: 30 Minutes | **Serves:** 6]

Ingredients:

- 1/2 stick unsalted butter
- 1/2 teaspoon vanilla extract
- 1/2 teaspoon ground cinnamon
- 2-ounces baker's chocolate, unsweetened.
- 2 tablespoons heavy cream
- 1/2 cup powdered erythritol
- A pinch of freshly grated nutmeg
- A pinch of pinch salt
- 2 eggs
- 1 cup almond flour

Directions:

1. Start by preheating your Air Fryer to 340 degrees F. Line a muffin tin with paper liners
2. In a mixing bowl, thoroughly combine all of the above ingredients. Scrape the batter into the cups
3. Bake for 11 minutes or until a skewer inserted into the middle of your muffin comes out dry. Transfer to a wire rack to cool for 15 to 20 minutes before unmolding
4. Arrange on a serving plate. Serve and enjoy!

Nutrition Information: 330 Calories; 21.5g Fat; 9.2g Carbs; 7.8g Protein; 2g Sugars

Old-Fashioned Fruit Tart

[Prep + Cook Time: 30 Minutes | **Serves:** 8]

Ingredients:

- 1 cup almond flour
- 1/3 cup vegetable shortening
- 1/4 cup powdered erythritol
- 4 tablespoons evaporated milk
- 1 teaspoon apple pie spice mix
- 1 cup cherries
- 1/3 cup almonds, chopped
- 1/4 teaspoon crystallized ginger
- A pinch of salt

Directions:

1. Start by preheating your Air Fryer to 360 degrees F
2. Combine the flour and vegetable shortening until the mixture is evenly crumbly. Now, stir in the powdered erythritol. Next, pour in the milk and mix until the dough is moist enough to hold together when you squeeze it.
3. Divide the dough into two balls. Now, roll out the dough ball to make a "pastry shell" and fill your pan. Now, trim the edges so they overlap the rim of the pan by 1-inch all the way around
4. Add the cherries and almonds. Sprinkle them with apple pie spice mix, crystallized ginger, and salt.
5. Roll out other ball and top your pie. Dot the top with the diced butter
6. Bake for 20 minutes or until thoroughly cooked. Remove your tart to a wire rack to cool completely. Serve and enjoy!

Nutrition Information: 191 Calories; 17.2g Fat; 8.1g Carbs; 4.4g Protein; 3.5g Sugars

Keto Almond Meringue Cookies

[Prep + Cook Time: 45 Minutes | **Serves:** 4]

Ingredients:

- 8 Egg Whites
- 2 teaspoon Lemon Juice
- 1½ teaspoon Vanilla Extract
- 1/2 teaspoon Almond Extract
- Melted Dark Chocolate to drizzle.
- 1 ⅓ cup Granulated Stevia
- 1/4 teaspoon Salt

Directions:

1. In a mixing bowl, add the egg whites, salt, and lemon juice. Beat using an electric mixer until foamy
2. Slowly add the stevia and continue beating until completely combined
3. Add the almond and vanilla extracts. Beat until stiff peaks form and glossy
4. Line a round baking sheet with parchment paper, that fits into the fryer basket

5. Fill a piping bag with the meringue mixture and pipe as many mounds on the baking sheet as you can leave 2-inch spaces between each mound
6. Place the baking sheet in the fryer basket and bake at 250°F for 5 minutes.
7. Reduce the temperature to 220°F and bake for 15 more minutes. The, reduce the temperature once more to 190°F and cook for 15 minutes
8. Remove the baking sheet and let the meringues cool for about 2 hours. Drizzle with the dark chocolate before serving

Nutrition Information: Calories: 34; Total Fat: 6g; Sodium: 25mg; Total Carbs: 1g; Net Carbs: 1g; Protein: 1.61g

Chocolate Soufflé

[**Prep + Cook Time:** 40 Minutes | **Serves:** 2]

Ingredients:
- 3 oz. Unsweetened Chocolate
- 1/4 cup Monk Fruit Sugar + more for garnishing
- 4 large Egg Whites
- 1 tablespoon Melted Butter
- 1 tablespoon Unmelted Butter
- 1/4 teaspoon Vanilla Extract
- 2 large Egg Yolks, at room temperature
- 1½ tablespoon Almond Flour

Directions:
1. Coat 2 6-oz ramekins with melted butter
2. Add the monk fruit sugar and swirl it in the ramekins to coat the butter. Pour out the remaining sugar and keep it
3. Melt the unmelted butter with the chocolate in a microwave and set aside.
4. In another bowl, beat the egg yolks vigorously. Add the vanilla and kept sugar. Beat to incorporate fully.
5. Add the chocolate mixture and mix well
6. Add the almond flour and mix it with no lumps
7. Preheat the Air Fryer to 330°F.
8. Whisk the egg whites in another bowl till it holds stiff peaks
9. Add 1/3 of the egg whites into the chocolate mixture and fold in gently and evenly
10. Share the mixture into the ramekins with ½ inch space left at the top. Place the ramekins in the fryer basket, close the Air Fryer and cook for 14 minutes. Dust with the remaining monk fruit sugar and serve.

Nutrition Information: Calories: 320; Total Fat: 25g; Sodium: 60mg; Total Carbs: 3.06g; Net Carbs: 3.01g; Protein: 11g

Christmas Mint Chocolate Cake

[**Prep + Cook Time:** 20 Minutes | **Serves:** 10]

Ingredients:
- 1 cup almond flour
- 1/2 cup coconut flour
- 1 ½ teaspoons baking powder
- 1/2 teaspoon kosher salt
- 3 tablespoons double cream
- 1/2 teaspoon mint extract
- 1 ½ cups powdered erythritol
- 2 tablespoons raw cocoa powder
- 1 stick butter
- 2 eggs
- 1-ounce baking chocolate, chopped into chunks

Directions:
1. Begin by preheating your Air Fryer to 360 degrees F. Lightly grease a baking pan
2. In a mixing bowl, thoroughly combine the flour, baking powder, and salt. Add powdered erythritol and cocoa; mix to combine
3. Cut in the butter and stir again.
4. In another bowl, mix the eggs with double cream; add this mixture to the bowl with the flour mixture

5. Lastly, add mint extract and chocolate; mix to combine well. Scrape the batter into the prepared baking pan
6. Bake for 10 minutes or until a skewer inserted into the middle of your cake comes out dry. Serve and enjoy!

Nutrition Information: 214 Calories; 17.1g Fat; 4.5g Carbs; 3.6g Protein; 2.3g Sugars

Crème Brulee

[Prep + Cook Time: 1 hour 10 Minutes | **Serves:** 3]

Ingredients:
- 1 cup Whipped Cream
- 2 Vanilla Pods
- 1 cup Milk
- 10 Egg Yolks
- 4 tablespoon Swerve Sugar + extra for topping

Directions:
1. In a pan, add the milk and cream. Cut the vanilla pods open and scrape the seeds into the pan with the vanilla pods also
2. Place the pan over medium heat on a stove top until almost boiled while stirring regularly. Turn off the heart.
3. Add the egg yolks to a bowl and beat it. Add the sugar and mix well but not too frothy
4. Remove the vanilla pods from the milk mixture and pour the mixture onto the eggs mixture while stirring constantly. Let it sit for 25 minutes
5. Fill 2 to 3 ramekins with the mixture. Place the ramekins in the fryer basket and cook them at 190°F for 50 minutes.
6. Once ready, remove the ramekins and let sit to cool
7. Sprinkle the remaining swerve sugar over and use a torch to melt the sugar, so it browns at the top.

Nutrition Information: Calories: 404; Total Fat: 32.15g; Sodium: 38mg; Total Carbs: 3.25g; Net Carbs: 3.25g; Protein: 4.06g

Best Ever Zucchini Cake

[Prep + Cook Time: 40 Minutes | **Serves:** 8]

Ingredients:
- 1 1/4 cups coconut flour
- 1 ½ teaspoons baking powder
- 2 eggs
- 1 zucchini
- 1/3 teaspoon cardamom
- 1/2 teaspoon salt
- 4 tablespoons coconut oil
- 1/2 cup erythritol
- 1/2 teaspoon ground star anise

For the Frosting:
- 2-ounces cream cheese
- 1 tablespoon butter, softened
- 1/2 cup powdered erythritol
- 2 tablespoons milk

Directions:
1. Start by preheating the Air Fryer to 325 degrees F for 5 minutes. Now, brush a baking pan with a butter-flavored nonstick cooking spray
2. In a mixing dish, thoroughly combine coconut flour with baking powder and salt
3. Beat coconut oil and erythritol until the mixture is smooth and uniform. Stir in the eggs and zucchini; mix again to combine well.
4. Add the flour mixture, along with cardamom and anise. Mix again
5. Spoon the batter into the baking pan. Transfer to the preheated Air Fryer and bake for 35 minutes. Transfer to a wire rack to cool completely
6. Meanwhile, make the frosting by mixing the remaining ingredients. Frost your cake and enjoy!

Nutrition Information: 133 Calories; 12.6g Fat; 5.1g Carbs; 3.2g Protein; 1.5g Sugars

Winter Fruit and Nut Dessert

[Prep + Cook Time: 45 Minutes | **Serves:** 5]

Ingredients:

- 1/2 teaspoon ground cinnamon
- 3 teaspoons coconut oil, cold
- 2 cups blueberries
- 1/2 cup walnuts, ground
- 3/4 cup swerve
- 1 cup heavy cream
- Nonstick cooking spray

Directions:

1. Begin by preheating your Air Fryer to 370 degrees F. Lightly spritz a baking pan with a nonstick cooking oil.
2. Now, add a layer of blueberries. Sprinkle with walnuts, swerve, and cinnamon; repeat until you run out of ingredients
3. Crumb the coconut oil over the top and bake for 35 minutes or until syrupy. Allow it to sit at room temperature until it is firm enough to slice
4. Serve at room temperature, topped with heavy cream. Serve and enjoy!

Nutrition Information: 155 Calories; 12.6g Fat; 9.1g Carbs; 2.8g Protein; 5.2g Sugars

Heavenly Chocolate Cake

[Prep + Cook Time: 25 Minutes | **Serves:** 8]

Ingredients:

- 1/2 cup erythritol, powdered
- 1 stick butter, at room temperature
- 2 eggs, beaten
- 1/8 teaspoon salt
- 1/8 teaspoon grated nutmeg
- 2-ounces unsweetened baker's chocolate
- 1 tablespoon heavy cream
- 1 cup almond flour
- 1 teaspoon baking powder
- 2 teaspoons raw cocoa powder
- 1/2 teaspoon vanilla essence
- 1/4 cup fresh raspberries, to decorate

Directions:

1. Begin by preheating your Air Fryer to 320 degrees F. Spritz the inside of a baking pan with a nonstick cooking spray
2. Now, beat the erythritol and butter with an electric mixer until the mixture is creamy. Fold in the eggs and mix again
3. Then, add the flour, baking powder, cocoa powder, vanilla, salt, and nutmeg. Afterwards, stir in chocolate and heavy cream; mix to combine well.
4. Scrape the batter into the prepared baking pan and level the surface using a spatula
5. Bake for 16 minutes or until a tester inserted in the center of your cake comes out dry. Decorate with fresh raspberries, cut into slices, and enjoy!

Nutrition Information: 185 Calories; 15.9g Fat; 8.5g Carbs; 6.4g Protein; 1.9g Sugars

Made in the USA
San Bernardino, CA
14 March 2019